Mastering the Law
of Attraction

Your Personal Change Blueprint

Debbie Taylor

Mastering the Law of Attraction

Your Personal Change Blueprint

Debbie Taylor

Disclaimer - Names, characters, businesses, events, and incidents are the products of the author's imagination. Any resemblance to actual persons, living or dead, or actual events is purely coincidental.

The information in this book, including the hypnosis recording, is NOT meant to replace medical or psychological treatment or consultation. If you have a serious medical condition, please consult with your physician.

Mastering the Law of Attraction

Your Personal Change Blueprint

Debbie Taylor

https://debbietaylor-author.com

ISBN - 978-1-7367549-0-0

First Printing: May 2021

Debbie Taylor
Intuitive Life Coach LLC
Portland, Oregon

https://intuitivelifecoachpublishing.com

Debbie Taylor is available to speak at your business or conference event on a variety of topics. Call 503-312-4660 for booking information.

Why Read This Book

What if I told you that you have been unsuccessful when it comes to manifesting your heart's desire because you have been sending out vibrational frequencies from two different, and often competing sources, your conscious mind, and your subconscious mind?

You are holding in your hands the secret to manifesting anything you choose. In this book, you will learn how to create a coherent flow of energy from both your conscious and subconscious mind and then focus that energy using your Personal Change Blueprint, which will manifest positive change in all areas of your life. Practicing your Personal Change Blueprint daily using self-hypnosis, following my easy-to-follow instructions, eliminates competing energy streams getting in the way of manifesting a joyful existence. No subject is off-limits! You can ...

- Build financial abundance
- Secure healthy relationships
- Find the perfect career
- Buy a house
- Get a new car
- Have a baby

And more!

Other books by Debbie Taylor

Are you interested in manifesting a lot of money? Follow along in Debbie's upcoming book, ***Mastering the Law of Attraction for Financial Abundance Your Personal Change Blueprint,*** for detailed instructions and examples on how to create your Personal Change Blueprint to manifest financial abundance.

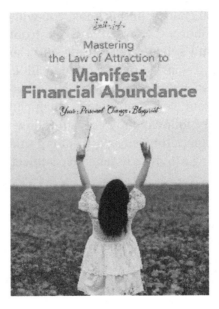

Scheduled for release Fall of 2021

Written by a leading expert with over thirty years experience as a hypnotist, speaker, author, online course creator, and teacher of manifesting with the Law of Attraction.

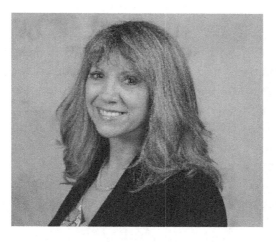

As a retired educator and administrator in both the public and private sectors, Debbie has spent her life teaching others how to create real, permanent change, in all areas of life. Combining her skill and love of hypnosis with her eight-step Personal Change Blueprint, Debbie has discovered the recipe for real-time manifestation.

As a lifelong student of spirituality, it didn't take long for her to make the connection between the microcosm of the subconscious mind and the macrocosm of universal energy and the workings of the Law of Attraction. Debbie's ability to explain how to make the Law of Attraction work goes beyond any other explanation available. The secret to manifesting is no longer a secret!

Do you want Debbie Taylor to be the motivational speaker at your next event?

Call 503-312-4660 or email Debbie at dtaylor@debbietaylor-author.com

Debbie's ability to explain the mechanics of the conscious and subconscious mind makes for an informative and entertaining experience for all attendees. Audience members are captivated as they learn not only how they acquire the subconscious programs that result in daily habits, rituals, and routines, but how they can put themselves in the driver's seat of the subconscious mind to eliminate unwanted thoughts and habits in exchange for the satisfaction of taking control of their lives in every area.

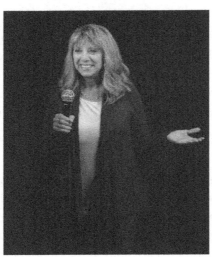

What others are saying about this book

Debbie takes a very ethereal concept and makes it a relatable 3D tangible reality. Following her method is a smooth path to the successes you want to experience in life.

Lynda Schumacher
President of Let's Talk Australia

...the best part with this book, technique, and hypnosis, in general, is that they are all respectful of your time and intelligence. The exercises are short and focused on your goals. The effects are tangible without anyone having to convince you of them. If you are receptive (and most of the population is), you don't have to take anyone's word for it; you can just experience them.

Daniel Cazan

The language is clear, concise and provides an important step-by-step process for changing beliefs and building a positive and powerful self-image. It recognizes the important connection between conscious decisions made by an individual - decisions that form our attitudes and expectations - and the unconscious mechanisms which respond to them. In particular, it provides a blueprint for change.

Ivan Kelly

Debbie's words in describing the law of attraction and the subconscious mind are simply put for anyone to be able to understand. As many people do not really understand the subconscious this book ties it all together in a very simple and easy to comprehend form.

Danny Picard

Table of Contents

"Decide what you want to be, do, and have, think the thoughts of it, emit the frequency, and your vision will become your life."
Rhonda Byrne, *The Secret*

Introduction

The Law of Attraction states: that which is like unto itself is drawn. As humans, we emit vibrational frequencies based on our thoughts, words, and emotions. Frequencies carry information. This is how we manifest relationships, careers, health, finances, opportunities, the communities we live in, and so on. The information riding on these frequencies is emitted out into the field. It aligns with matching frequencies and brings back to us the manifestations we know as our life experience, relationships, financial status, career opportunities, and so on.

What if I told you that you send out vibrational frequencies from two different parts, your conscious mind, and your subconscious mind? The information riding on the frequency of your conscious mind typically reflects what you are focused on in the present moment and contains the dreams and aspirations you want for yourself in the here and now. For those who consciously work to manifest abundance in your life, you are sending out positive intentions from your conscious mind.

Here's the problem. When looking at the totality of the frequency you are sending out, only 1-5% of it comes from the conscious part of your mind. The rest, 95% of that frequency, is coming from your subconscious mind. The subconscious part of your mind is where you house your habits, rituals, routines, beliefs, values, memories, and more. I call this the grand archives of your past. The information contained on this frequency is old news. Until you update the information in the subconscious part of your mind, you will continue to manifest life experiences that reflect your past no matter how many vision boards you make, how many pretty words you say, or how many times you smudge your house.

The Law of Attraction is real, and it's simple to understand that the reason you have not been able to manifest what you want in your life is that the dominant frequency you are emitting is coming from the subconscious part of your mind. The conscious part of your mind is the part you are using when you deliberately focus on what you want. Still, if you don't know how to get that 1-5% of your desire to match what the subconscious part of your mind is emitting, you will continue to experience the absence of what you want.

I have been a professional hypnotist for years. My clients may not realize it, but when they come to me for help to lose weight or quit smoking, what they are asking me to do is help them manifest a new way of life, as in "make the Law of Attraction work for me and program my subconscious mind to send out the frequency of what I want instead of what I don't want."

After years of explaining this process to one client at a time, I thought it would be helpful to share this information in a book. So here it is, *Mastering the Law of Attraction Your Personal Change Blueprint*. Using my eight-step process with self-hypnosis will allow you to reprogram your subconscious mind, thus aligning the frequencies of your conscious mind with your subconscious mind. This is how you master the Law of Attraction to manifest the life of your dreams. When it comes to mastering the Law of Attraction using your Personal Change Blueprint, no subject is off-limits. You are a limitless creator!

I am passionate about spreading this information to as many people as I can. It is so important to me that people understand they are not broken, that happiness is not just for other people, that every one of us can manifest the kind of life we want for ourselves. All you need to learn is how to align the stream of energy from your subconscious mind with the stream of energy focused on by your conscious mind. Developing your Personal Change Blueprint will create the road map, and self-hypnosis will set your plan into action.

I will walk you through the process step by step. We start by identifying precisely what you want to manifest and then examine the potential payoffs for not having what you want in the first place. These payoffs live at the subconscious level and are often the barrier preventing you from accomplishing your goals. Most of us are unaware of these subconscious payoffs because they are subconscious, below the level of awareness. By addressing the perceived obstacles and payoffs at the subconscious level, we can thank them, bless them, and send them on their way.

Once you have cleared the path and identified your desired outcome, you will be ready to build your Personal Change Blueprint. I will guide you toward identifying the changes you will notice from the perspective of having manifested your desire. There will be evidence. I will show you how to identify what that manifestation looks like, sounds like, and feels like. Together we will take a look at this beautiful blueprint you are creating, and I will help you understand what having this manifestation does for you. How does this enhance your well-being? You will create imagery of how this manifestation influences your relationships, career and finances, health, self-esteem, and how it will expand your spiritual practice. You will create a beautiful mind movie of your life as you would have it, in every detail.

By reviewing your Personal Change Blueprint daily using self-hypnosis, you will not only be rewiring your brain physically, but you will also be communicating and emitting a congruent vibrational frequency into the universe about what you want to manifest as if you already have it. This is how you learn to align your frequencies, conscious and subconscious, to send out a very clear, coherent request into the universe. This is how you master the Law of Attraction using your Personal Change Blueprint!

I am thrilled that you have purchased this book. Not because I want to sell more books but because I know that if you follow my instructions, you will experience manifestations beyond anything you have ever experienced before. I use self-hypnosis every day, and my life is amazing! That doesn't mean my life is free of conflict or that I don't have more desires to manifest. I will always find something more to want. But what a blessing to understand how to remove the obstacles in the form of outdated subconscious programs that can keep me pinned down to an unhappy existence. Now I am able to take control of the frequency I am emitting. It is true that if you change your thoughts, you change your life, but you have to change those thoughts at both the conscious and subconscious levels.

The Personal Change Blueprint you will learn in this book has proven results. Each chapter provides clear instructions with examples to give you the opportunity to master the Law of Attraction. Why wait? There is a universe of well-being and abundance out there just waiting for you!

To get you started, I have provided a relaxation MP3 for you to listen to every day. This recording will wire your brain to go into hypnosis so that your self-hypnosis experience will be optimal. Listening to this recording is the first step in mastering the Law of Attraction using your Personal Change Blueprint. You can get your free download here: https://debbietaylor-author.com/free-audio01

"You have to begin to tell the story of your life as you now want it to be and discontinue the tales of how it has been or of how it is."
Abraham Hicks

Chapter One

What Are You Wired to Experience?

Manifesting your greatest desire for abundance is easy, but only if your brain is wired for it. Do you realize that everything you do is possible only because your brain is wired to do it?

When I say "wired," what I mean is that you have neural pathways in your brain that light up or get activated when you decide to do something. This applies to everything you do, from the way you pick up a fork, reach for a doorknob, drive your car, scratch your head, or tie your shoes. All your habits, rituals, routines, beliefs, values, memories, and more are represented physically in your brain as neural pathways. Every time you put on your running shoes, the ones with laces, your "shoe tying" neural pathways are stimulated, allowing you to tie those shoes without giving it a second thought. If, for some reason, those neural pathways were damaged or severed, you would not for the life of you remember how to tie your shoes.

A great wine connoisseur has been trained in detecting the subtle characteristics of the wines they are tasting. Their brains are wired to taste and smell these differences. Mine is not. A musician is trained and experienced to detect the sound of an instrument that is slightly out of tune or to notice the sound of a drum that is somewhat offbeat. Their brains are wired to hear the differences. Mine is not. Hunters are taught to see a herd of deer on a hillside miles away. Their brains are wired to see those animals from a great distance. Mine is not. However, if I so desired, I could wire my brain or create the habit of doing any of the above examples. It just takes focus, desire, and repetition to wire my brain to be different than it is, to create new neural pathways that allow me to taste, see, or hear like a pro. In this book, I am going to teach you how to wire your brain to perceive abundance. Mine is. But first, let's talk more about neural pathways.

Neural Pathways

Where do these neural pathways come from, can we make more, and how much say do we have regarding the content of these neural pathways?

When we are born, we are like a new computer that comes pre-loaded with all kinds of programs, all in the form of neural pathways. These are our instincts, our reflexes, our mannerisms, and more. As we grow and learn, our brain continues to grow and learn, and the number of neural pathways expands exponentially as we observe and absorb everything in our environment. As we continue to live out our lives, we identify various interests, and we consciously choose to learn new things. Every time we learn something new, we add to the tremendous number of neural pathways in our brains as we enrich our lives.

However, we cannot perceive anything we are not wired to perceive. For example, dog brains are wired to hear sounds that we cannot hear. Eagles have brains that are wired such that they can see great distances. While we may or may not have the ability to rewire our brains to hear what a dog hears or to see like an eagle, we *can* wire our brains for abundance in all areas of our lives.

Think about a house and the wiring in that house. Depending on when this house was built, it was wired to meet the needs of the homeowners at the time of construction. A home built in 1920 is going to have very different wiring than a home built in 2020. At the time of construction, the needs of the inhabitants in these two homes are very different. Thinking of myself as a house built in 1957, I can guarantee you that the wiring I came with is not sufficient to meet my needs now. And so, I update my wiring, or in this case my neural pathways, by creating habits (including thought habits), rituals, routines, beliefs, values, and memories that are a more accurate reflection of who I am right here, right now, in this present moment.

The configuration of our wiring creates emotional and behavioral programs specific to each of us. We all have a lot of programming. Here's the difficulty: these programs do not update themselves on their own, just like an old house doesn't rewire itself. These programs are just that—programs. They are very impersonal. They do not care if you love them or hate them, or if they will make you healthy or make you sick. For many people, the programs running their lives are old, outdated, and not necessarily relevant to today's situation. You can only perceive what you are wired to perceive. You owe it to yourself and your loved ones to update your wiring regularly, so your reactions and responses to life events are an accurate reflection of what is going on in your life in the present moment.

If you feel you are *not* wired for abundance, keep reading because I am going to teach you how to change that. Learning how to rewire your brain is easy. The method I use will make more sense if you learn a few things about how your brain works beforehand.

Conscious and Subconscious

This brings us to a discussion about the conscious and subconscious parts of your mind.

The conscious part of you is the *you* that is reading this book. This part of you houses your creativity, volition, and ability to compare, contrast, and analyze things. It is the conscious part of you that is awake, alive, and consciously aware that you exist.

Your subconscious mind is your habit mind. Once you have learned something, wanted or not, it gets stored away into the grand warehouse of your subconscious. This is the part of your mind that houses all your habits, rituals, routines, beliefs, values, memories, and all those programs.

Take a moment and think about these two parts of you and see if you can figure out which one is running the show. In other words, what percentage of your day would you say you are *consciously* aware of what you are doing? Here is the answer: from the moment you wake up to the moment you fall back to sleep at night, you are only consciously aware of 1-5% of what is going on in your day. That is not a typo. You are only consciously aware of what you are doing 1-5% of your day; that's only 5% of the day—on your best day! You can see how important it is to make sure your subconscious mind is running current and relevant programs that serve you in the present moment.

When I tell my clients they are only consciously aware of 1-5% of their day, I make sure they understand that my goal is not to increase that percentage. My goal is to help them realize that if the subconscious part of their mind runs the show 95-99% of the time, then it's in their best interest to figure out how to access that part of their mind and update those habits.

Most habits are good. They make it easy for us to function without having to re-learn everything we do. But, unless you intentionally update your habits, the older you get, the more distance (often showing up as conflict) there is between who you are now (acting the way you want to act) and the behavioral habits you engage in (which may be very outdated and out of sync).

You may already be understanding that although your conscious mind is ready and willing, it is your *subconscious* mind that is running the show. This is an excellent time to shift gears for a moment and talk about how the Law of Attraction works. You'll see how this all ties together shortly.

The Law of Attraction

What does it mean to say that we "attract" things into our lives? When we look at the unwanted aspects of our lives, it is crazy to think that we would ever intentionally attract such misery. To understand this better, you have to realize that we all emit a vibrational frequency. This is a fact. It is science. Think of yourself as a human radio. You are both a sender and a receiver of vibrational frequencies specific to you, and these frequencies carry information.

Radio waves are measured in hertz. You have probably seen images depicting radio waves. They are a series of repeating peaks and valleys. The entire pattern is called a cycle, and the number of cycles, or times it repeats itself in a second, is called a frequency. Do you know call numbers on radio stations like 98.1 or 103.5? Those numbers represent the specific frequency or the number of times a particular cycle repeats itself in one second. Different frequencies carry different information. Radio stations have the technology to put specific information on specific frequencies and send it out into the air. Your radio has the technology to access multiple frequencies, bringing you a variety of stations to listen to.

Now realize that we do the same thing with our energy; we are both senders and receivers of frequencies. As we send out our specific frequencies, they go out and find matching frequencies with matching information and bring it back to us. This is how the Law of Attraction works. It is really quite impersonal. We simply attract information in the form of wealth or poverty, good health or illness, relationships, jobs, religious beliefs, opportunities, experiences, and more based on the frequency we are emitting. The Law of Attraction does not punish or reward us; it simply reflects back to us what we are emitting in terms of frequency. Easy enough to understand, right?

If you have negative programming about abundance at the subconscious level, and most of us do, then all the consciously positive words in the world will not change your lot in life because your conscious mind is only contributing 1-5% of the vibration you are emitting. Most people are unable to make the Law of Attraction work for them because they do not know how to reprogram those neural pathways from the past—all those programs of poverty consciousness, jealousy, fear of success, the evilness of money, and so on. It is that subconscious state of mind that is sending out your requests to the universe. What is *your* subconscious emitting? If you see wealthy people as rude, arrogant snobs, then you are bringing into your life experience more exposure to rich people who you see as rude, arrogant snobs. If you are worried about not having enough money to pay your bills, you will bring back into your life the experience of not having enough money to pay your bills. If you are feeling left out and isolated, then you are asking for more of the same.

Understand that even if your conscious mind is doing all the right things, it is only a small part of what is going on. Your subconscious mind dictates what you are doing and saying, along with how you react or respond. Your subconscious mind is emitting the dominant frequency, and if the information on this frequency is not wired for abundance, you will not attract or experience abundance.

I want to clarify that the term "abundance" here reflects abundance in all areas, not just money. Money is one of the more common desires of those wanting to learn more about the Law of Attraction, but it also refers to an abundance of health, happiness, well-being, love, career fulfillment, self-esteem, relationships, friendships, laughter, freedom, opportunity, adventure, and so on.

Imagine the frequency you are sending out into the cosmos, like ordering from a menu at the Universal Restaurant of Abundance. If you go through this menu of life and do nothing but point out what you do *not* want, or everything you see that bugs you, even things you hate, your server has no idea what you want. You will be served what you focused on. You emit the frequency of whatever you are focused on—the good, the bad, and the ugly.

I will teach you how to change this frequency using self-hypnosis to reinforce your Personal Change Blueprint so that your conscious mind and your subconscious mind can order off the same menu.

I use the Law of Attraction with every client I work with. I don't necessarily use the phrase Law of Attraction, but that is what I do. I help people create the habit of living a different reality in the privacy of their minds to create new neural pathways. By practicing hypnosis regularly, either by listening to one of my recordings or practicing self-hypnosis, brand new neural pathways are created based on what the client wants to change, leading to concrete manifestations of the desired outcome.

Here is a story about Bob, a guy wanting to rewire his brain to manifest some freedom from depression and anxiety.

The Story of Bob

Bob was beside himself with despair. He had severe depression that was creating extreme anxiety and daily panic attacks. His doctor wanted to increase his dose of antidepressants; a suggestion Bob adamantly opposed. His desired outcome was to free himself from the depression, anxiety, and panic attacks that had become his constant companions so that he could stop taking the medications altogether. He thought maybe hypnosis could help him.

As a hypnotist, I want to make the point that I never suggest that clients begin or cease taking any medication. I am not qualified or interested in making that call. In a situation like Bob's, I always insist that my clients work with their medical doctor to either begin or stop taking any medication. Let's get back to Bob's story.

Bob's story began about five years before his hypnosis session. He was happily married; he and his wife were both gainfully employed, had the house of their dreams, no kids by choice. Life was good. Unfortunately, his wife got sick and was diagnosed with cancer. They both did all the things the doctors tell you to do in this situation, but sadly, her cancer worsened. It was not long until she was so sick, she had to quit her job. Bob started staying home more and more often to care for her, and soon he lost his job. She suffered a long, sad, heart-wrenching death, and by the time it was over, Bob had lost his wife, job, home, and now his mental and emotional stability. The local community stepped in to help. Bob was offered a job at a local business as a janitor. He gladly took the job and went to work every day, going through all the motions of someone living a normal life.

At work, Bob was starting to notice an increase in his anxiety symptoms anytime one of the other employees would try to strike up a conversation with him. He began isolating himself to avoid feelings of anxiety. He did anything he could to avoid the panic attacks that had begun. Bob was stuck. All he could think about was his loss, his sadness, his depression, his absolute lack of interest in anything. He had considered suicide several times but had promised his wife he would never kill himself. Bob was at his wit's end by the time he found his way into my office.

After our initial meeting, a four-session course of treatment was recommended for Bob. He came in for his first appointment, and I helped him identify what he truly wanted. By creating a Personal Change Blueprint for Bob, we described what his outcome looked like, sounded like, felt like, and so on.

The hypnosis part of his session was recorded so that he could listen to the suggestions daily for two weeks until his second appointment. As clients listen to their hypnosis session audio recordings while in a state of hypnosis, they begin to create a mind movie of how life *could* be, how they would like it to be. Bob was feeling better and making progress by the time he came in for his second session. He had listened to his hypnosis recording daily, as instructed, and was beginning to rewire his brain for happiness.

The journey this man had been on over the previous five years was a journey of fear, loss, sadness, grief, depression, anxiety, and more. For *five* years, he lived with these states of being and had started feeling worse by the day.

At Bob's second appointment with me, a new recording was made based on his progress as we focused on his next steps. Again, he was instructed to listen to this new recording each day until his third session.

Bob called me a few days before his third appointment and asked if he could have a refund for the remaining sessions. He said he was fine, back to normal, feeling great again, and was certain that if he had just waited a few more weeks, everything would have settled down—just a few more weeks.

I was astonished that Bob did not realize it was the hypnosis helping him. He believed that he would have been fine after *five years* of suffering had he just waited a few more weeks. I encouraged Bob to finish up with his package of four sessions. He came in for one more, begrudgingly, and then forfeited the fourth session.

It was exciting that Bob had responded so well to hypnosis. He manifested freedom from so many things he no longer wanted to experience. Even though he had been suffering for over five years, and things had been getting worse before he started hypnosis, he was happy again. I still laugh when I think of him saying, "If I'd just waited a few more weeks, I'm sure things would have been fine." I did not *need* him to believe that it was the hypnosis that helped him. What I cared about was that he was feeling better.

By listening to his hypnosis recordings daily, Bob's subconscious mind created a whole new neighborhood of neural pathways. He was a particularly good subject, and subsequently, his daily life experience reflected his updated wiring. The content of Bob's recordings, based on his Personal Change Blueprint, aligned his subconscious mind with his conscious focus of feeling better. This is a significant example of how the Law of Attraction works.

It's essential to know that the Law of Attraction is always at work, not just when you are using it for things you *want*. Everything in your life is the way it is because of the Law of Attraction. It is like the Law of Gravity; it works all the time, not just when you want your shoes to stay on the floor.

How can you tell what you are manifesting with the Law of Attraction? Just look at your life. How is your health? How are your finances, your relationships, your career, or your spiritual practice? Every detail of your life is the way it is because you have been sending out a particular frequency, and the majority of the frequencies we send out, 95-99% of them, are coming from the subconscious mind. We do not realize what we are sending out at the subconscious level because it is below conscious awareness. Your situation in life reflects the vibrational frequency you emit at both the conscious and subconscious levels, but mainly at the subconscious level.

We get what we focus on whether we want it or not. If you focus on not having enough money, you will continue not to have enough money. If you focus, or ruminate, on the negative traits of your ex-spouse, you will draw those same traits right back to you in your next relationship. If you focus on what lousy drivers there are in your town, you will see lousy drivers everywhere you go. What are you focusing on that you want more or less of?

Now that you understand more about how the Law of Attraction *really* works, and you understand that your subconscious mind is sending out the dominant frequency responsible for what is going on in your life, you are likely to be more than ready to learn how to access your subconscious mind so you can program its frequency to match the frequency of your conscious mind. This is how to master the Law of Attraction, and this is what I will teach you to do using self-hypnosis to set your Personal Change Blueprint into action.

Self-hypnosis is an excellent way to create the subconscious habit of focusing on what you want, all day, every day. Going into a hypnotic trance is easy. We do it all the time. It is a natural state of being. However, knowing what to do once you are in that state of hypnosis is the most important part of the process. I will share with you the step-by-step process, the Personal Change Blueprint, I use with my clients. It is easy, natural, and effective.

Please be aware that this is a hands-on approach. You will have to actively contribute some effort to apply the eight-step process that makes up your Personal Change Blueprint. It is the mastery of this process that will allow you to master the Law of Attraction.

In the next chapter, I will describe two particularly important facts about how you can learn to control the frequency sent out by your subconscious mind. The first is how to talk to the subconscious mind effectively and train it to focus on what you *do* want. The words you use are vitally important. Second, the subconscious mind does not know the difference between really doing something or just pretending or thinking about doing something. This can work for us or against us. I will teach you how to use this to your advantage.

"Man, alone, has the power to transform his thoughts into physical reality; man, alone, can dream and make his dreams come true."
Napoleon Hill

Chapter Two
Introduction to Your Personal
Change Blueprint

Years ago, a friend of mine saw the movie *The Secret*. Afterward, she was so excited and sure that her riches were just around the corner! She was on a high for about two weeks until she got tired of waiting for things to change. Like many others who had seen *The Secret*, she lost interest and gave up on the belief that you could get rich quickly just by thinking about being rich and constantly repeating, "I am wealthy, I am wealthy, I am wealthy."

It didn't take long until she concluded that the Law of Attraction was a myth and did not actually work. She did nothing more to find out why it didn't work for her, and I suppose, like most people, she had no idea where to look for answers. Look no further. In this book, you will learn the secret they left out of *The Secret*—the part that makes it work!

The Law of Attraction manifests through the thoughts coming from the conscious mind and the subconscious mind, but mostly the subconscious mind, by drawing to you thoughts and ideas of a matching frequency. Your manifestations come to you in the form of people who think like you, corresponding situations and circumstances, opportunities, and life experiences. It shows up by bringing people into your life that can help you with your plans. It shows up by creating situations and circumstances that match what you focus on, whether you want it or not. As you can tell, defining exactly what you want is essential.

Two Very Important Points

When it comes to the creation of new neural pathways, which in turn result in new habits, rituals, routines, and so on, there are two important facts to consider:

1. Your subconscious mind is like a computer in that it speaks its own language.

The language of the subconscious mind is imagery. All the incoming data that you receive through your five senses each day is translated into imagery. This imagery makes up the content of your subconscious programming. Please understand that your mind *cannot* picture you *not* doing something. In other words, it ignores words like won't, don't, stop, quit, and so on. If you tell yourself that you are going to *stop* smoking cigarettes after dinner each night, your mind actually creates an image of you smoking cigarettes. You have to figure out what you will be doing instead and focus on that. If you are not smoking cigarettes after dinner each night, then what are you doing? This would be the question to ask yourself if you were trying to quit smoking cigarettes after dinner each night.

In my opinion, this is one of the most important things to remember when it comes to retraining your subconscious mind. As humans, we are predestined to focus on the negative. In a different time and place far in the past, this inclination helped us survive. By focusing on potential dangers and external threats, we were able to stay out of danger and survive. In today's world, for most of us, there is no tiger lurking around the corner, no tribe ready to send a warring party around the bend to attack our village. Yet, we consistently talk and think about what we do not like, what we do not want, and what we think is wrong with everyone else. It is no wonder, so many of us have given up on being in control of our daily life experience. We continue to attract unwanted experiences in practically all areas of our lives.

As you continue to study this material and learn more about the Law of Attraction and self-hypnosis, you will naturally start paying more attention to the words you hear from others, becoming more aware of the words you use yourself, and more aware of the content of your thoughts. Listen, and then think about the imagery created by those words and thoughts. You may be surprised at how negatively focused our culture is. For example, if you want to lose weight, is your internal dialog about how badly you need to stop eating chips at night while watching television? What image does that create? If you want to sleep well at night, do you complain all day about how many hours you were awake the night before and how tired you are? What image does that create? If you want to stop biting your nails, do you look at them with disgust and tell yourself that you have got to stop biting your nails all the time? What image does that create? I think you are getting the point.

Your subconscious mind does not know the difference between the words you speak and the thoughts you think, so beware, my friends, you may be sabotaging yourself based on nothing more than thought habits. This brings me to the second most important thing I want you to know about your subconscious mind and how it either creates or reinforces programmed behavior in the form of neural pathways.

2. Your subconscious mind does not know the difference between really doing something or just pretending to do something.

By pretending, I mean thinking about it, talking about it, listening to it, watching it, and so on. Every day as I work with clients, they tell me about some traumatic event that happened years ago, and they begin sobbing as if the event were happening right at that moment. Notice your emotions the next time you are watching a scary movie. Even though your conscious mind knows it is just a movie, your subconscious mind responds as if the action in the movie were happening in real-time. Some movies are very anxiety-producing, as is the news. We use this to our advantage in self-hypnosis because we can create a mind movie depicting the future we want for ourselves. Through repetition, we can program the subconscious to make this mind movie become a reality through the development of new neural pathways.

When I work with clients, I often use a process called "future pacing." Future pacing allows us to practice an event the way we want it to be before it happens in reality. I use this for clients needing help with public speaking, test anxiety, social anxiety, and many other situations. By repeatedly practicing the event the way you want it to be while in a state of hypnosis, your brain creates new neural pathways. Those new neural pathways become new habits, rituals, and routines, and they begin to emit the vibrational frequency of what you want from the subconscious mind.

Whatever we are focused on is being practiced into reality. You are always practicing whatever your mind is focused on. Do you think you will get better sleep by focusing on *not* sleeping or *on* sleeping? Do you think you will create the habit of healthy eating by focusing on and practicing the idea of healthy eating, or by focusing on how much you hate being overweight and what a miserable wreck of a person you are because you cannot get it together?

You get what you focus on, and *that* is manifestation. What are you manifesting that is the opposite of what you want? Are you tir manifesting by default and ready to start manifesting by design? Then keep reading. Remember these two facts explained above. I will return to them often.

In the next chapter, we begin the journey of creating your Personal Change Blueprint. Your blueprint will become the roadmap to your mastery of the Law of Attraction. I will devote a chapter to each step and explain in detail, with examples, how to craft your suggestions for optimal success. You can find a list of the eight steps in Appendix A, or you can print off the free PDFs found on my website at https://debbietaylor-author.com/free-blueprint-pdf and get ready to change your life.

"Be thankful for what you have, you'll end up having more. If you concentrate on what you don't have, you will never ever have enough."
Oprah Winfrey

Chapter Three

Overview of the 8 Step Process – Your Personal Change Blueprint

B efore we explore the eight-step process of creating your Personal Change Blueprint, I want to outline each step ahead of time to help put this in perspective. The prerequisite to designing your Personal Change Blueprint is to choose a manifestation topic that is meaningful to you. It can be anything from getting a new car to getting into bed on time each night, keeping up on the housework, or anything in between. Choose something fun and easy at first to manifest and take your time filling out your Personal Change Blueprint.

In the chapters following, I explain each of the eight steps in more detail and provide examples of possible answers based on a hypothetical choice of either manifesting financial abundance, a healthy relationship, or a dream career.

Looking at examples of how other people have answered the questions in the eight-step Personal Change Blueprint will make it easier for you to understand how to create your own blueprint. If you happen to choose the same topic as any of the examples, personalize your answers. We could all choose the same topic to focus on, but our blueprints would all be different.

Step One – Your Payoffs and Your *Now* Statement

There is a belief that behind every behavior, there is a positive intention. I agree with this statement, but it deserves some explanation. Sometimes we have to look back in time to when a specific behavior was created to see what the positive intention was at the time the behavior became a habit.

For example, I started smoking cigarettes at a young age. By the time I was an adult and was ready to quit, there was no positive intention for the smoking habit, none at all. But, at the time the smoking behavior was established, it was full of positive intentions. It was fun! I loved hanging out with the older kids. It made me feel part of something, I was accepted, and I liked the rebelliousness of it as well. As an adult, there was no payoff, but there was an original payoff that was created at the time the behavior was established.

In step one, you will be asked to identify any possible positive intentions or payoffs related to the absence of what you want. These will be positive intentions that were, or could have been, relevant when your unwanted habit, behavior, or belief was established. These are the subconscious payoffs for maintaining that undesirable behavior. Remember, once a behavior is established and firmly rooted in your subconscious mind, it is boxed up and stored away. It does not keep pace with your personal growth and development. These payoffs can be decades old.

Once you have identified one or more possible payoffs for that unwanted behavior, you are ready to let your subconscious mind know that you appreciate that positive intention but that you are ready to thank it, bless it, and send it on its way.

This is where you craft your NOW statement. This is where you tell your subconscious mind that the past is over, things are changing regarding this behavior, and that *now this is how it's going to be.* You are explaining to your subconscious mind why you are willing to give up the payoff.

Perhaps you gained a lot of weight when you went through a divorce. The payoff from that bad habit was the comfort of eating yummy foods that took your mind off your troubles for a few minutes. You acknowledge your awareness of that payoff to your subconscious mind. You let it know that you appreciate its attempts at helping you. You acknowledge that "at that time" it was helpful, but *now*, you're ready to reclaim your health and to be free from the need to comfort yourself with food. The examples in the chapter on step one will help clarify this process and explain how others have answered this question.

Step Two –Crafting your Outcome for Exactly What You Want

If you were writing a story about your desired manifestation, this step could be the title of your story. Here you are identifying in a simple statement exactly what you want—not the *result* of having what you want, but what you actually want. This is an outcome statement. Many people think they want to lose weight but what they really want is to have a healthy relationship with food. Weight loss is the result of having what they want.

In the chapter explaining step two, I provide guidance and examples of possible outcome statements based on the choice to manifest either financial abundance, a healthy relationship, or your dream career. Again, these are examples intended to help you understand how to develop this part of your Personal Change Blueprint. Your answers will be specific to you and your topic. Your outcome statement must be a statement of what you want rather than what you don't want.

Step Three –Your Evidence

Once you reach this step, you will be answering the remaining questions, including this one, *as if* you had already accomplished your outcome, meaning you *have* manifested your desire. This is important. Here you get to practice your pretending skills to the max. I suggest that as you work your way through this Personal Change Blueprint, you go back to step two each time, re-read your outcome, then answer each question from the perspective of having already accomplished the outcome. Read it back to yourself in a way that sounds like this: "Because I have manifested (fill in the blank with your desired outcome), I notice (the evidence)." Or, "When I think about having this change in my life, I see (the evidence)." In step three, you will be identifying the evidence proving and demonstrating to you that you have, in fact, accomplished your outcome. What changes will you notice, what will be different? If you find yourself saying things like, "I'll have more energy," or "I'll be more productive," flesh that out a little more. What kinds of things will you be doing with that energy? What will you be accomplishing because you are more productive?

As you develop your Personal Change Blueprint, you will be creating a magnificent mind movie to review in self-hypnosis. Make it rich, colorful, and full of detail. The sky is the limit!

Step Four – Imagery Associated with Your Manifestation

In the chapter outlining step four, I will ask you to identify any imagery that comes to mind when you think of having accomplished your outcome. I will remind you later, but it's important to note that it's alright to repeat some of the information from one step to another. As you approach this part of your Personal Change Blueprint, you will ask yourself, "When I think of all the changes happening in my life because I have accomplished my outcome, I see ..." Your answers may be literal or figurative. If you see yourself on the hillside dancing in the sunlight, then so be it. The more time you spend focusing on the results of manifesting what you want, the more you stimulate ideas and images at the subconscious level. The more time you spend focusing on the results of manifesting what you want, the better you align the vibrational frequencies of your conscious and subconscious mind.

Step Five – Sounds Associated with Your Manifestation

Have you ever thought about the changing sounds in your environment once you have manifested something new in your life? If you are focused on the manifestation of a new vacuum or a new stereo, then the answer is probably yes. However, most of us don't pay much attention to sounds.

In step five of your Personal Change Blueprint, I will ask you to do just that. First, go back and review your outcome, repeat it to yourself a few times and then ask yourself what kind of sounds are associated with the manifestation of your outcome? If you are stuck on this one, I'll give you some hints. An associated sound could be the voice in your head, your internal dialog. It could be comments from other people, or it could be the absence of a particular sound. These sounds can be literal or figurative, and perhaps because you have manifested your outcome, you hear angels singing, or you hear the sigh of relief. Those are perfectly good answers.

Step Six – Feelings Associated With Your Manifestation

In step six, I want you to connect with the emotional and physical feelings you notice because you have manifested your outcome. When you look back at the answers, you filled out in your Personal Change Blueprint, and if you are like most of us, you will notice that many of your answers describe feelings. Not to worry, you don't have to transfer those details to the "feeling" section; just add the new ones. If you feel free, describe what you feel free to do. If you feel happy, describe what you are happy about. If your body feels better because you manifest better health, describe how good it feels and what a relief it is to be free from the old discomfort. That creates much better imagery than saying your feet aren't on fire anymore.

Step Seven – What Change Does for You

Your Personal Change Blueprint is coming along nicely by the time you reach step seven. Before you answer step seven, I will ask you to review all the information you have added to your Personal Change Blueprint so far. You may think of new ideas to add here and there. After you have reviewed your blueprint in its entirety, I want you to sit back and look at the big picture. Look at what you are creating. Look at the magnificence of this manifestation and all that comes with it, and then ask yourself what having this change will do for you.

If you were building a new home and you designed every square inch of it just the way you wanted it, what would having a new home built to your specifications do for you? Why is this manifestation important? What's the big deal about *this* manifestation? Take the time you need to reflect on this question. It is important.

Step Eight – Positive Influences on Your Relationships, Career/Finances, Health, Self-esteem, and Spirituality

At first glance, the questions in this eighth step seem like the questions in the preceding steps. But as you work your way through each step and allow yourself to mentally and emotionally experience the perspective of already having what you want, your creativity and imagination will start to flourish. You will notice that more and more details come to you at this stage, and it's perfectly fine to go back and add more information to any step you want.

I think of this last step as the domino effect. After all, you get to take a good look at how many things are going to improve because you are manifesting this one change in your life. And it's an all-positive change.

Step eight allows you to tie up any loose ends by identifying and describing the positive influences you will notice because you have manifested your outcome. Here you will be prompted to think about how your relationships will change, relationships with family, friends, coworkers, strangers, and so on. You will reflect on the positive influences you will notice regarding your career and finances. When you think of the changes in your health, you will see better emotional, physical, psychological, and intellectual health in many cases. Describe those in detail.

Perhaps the most significant positive influence will be on your self-esteem. How can you feel anything but proud of yourself for manifesting your outcome and realizing that you now have the key to manifesting anything you choose in any part of your life? And finally, if you have a spiritual practice, you may see a positive influence on the rituals and routines that you enjoy. If you do not have a spiritual practice, no worries, just leave this part blank.

When designing your Personal Change Blueprint to master the Law of Attraction, you can take as little or as much time as you want to complete your blueprint. I recommend taking a few hours and creating your blueprint in one sitting and then coming back to it after a few hours or a day and reviewing your answers. There is no hurry to any of this and if filling out one question every day or so works best for you, then do what is best for you.

> *"Most people are thinking about what they don't want, and they're wondering why it shows up over and over again."*
> John Assaraf

Chapter Four

Step One – Your Payoffs and Your *Now* Statement

As mentioned in the previous chapter, the prerequisite to step one is having identified the topic you want to manifest. It can be an object, a new habit, a belief, a new perspective, whatever you want. If this is your first time creating a Personal Change Blueprint, choose something light, something meaningful, and fun to work with. For example, maybe you want to manifest the habit of waking up at 5:30 AM every morning, heading to the gym and *enjoying* it. Maybe you want to manifest an object, like new dishes or a new skill saw. Once you are adept at designing your Personal Change Blueprint and have mastered the Law of Attraction on a regular basis, you can focus on the big-ticket desires without going off in the weeds about the absence of what you want. If you feel any sense of urgency or tension about the absence of whatever you are choosing to focus on, start with something more simple, more neutral. Once you have proven to yourself how easy it is to master the Law of Attraction, you'll be able to focus on those big-ticket items with ease.

Get comfortable, pen in hand, and let's get started.

Step one is about identifying the payoffs, the positive intentions behind the absence of what you want. In other words, what is, or was, the value or benefit of the problem? The following examples are intended to help you get an idea of how others have answered this question by looking at the payoff for not having financial abundance, the payoff for not having a healthy relationship, or the payoff for not having a dream career. What are the payoffs related to your specific situation? Remember, if you can't identify a payoff that is valid in the here and now, then the payoff was most likely created in the past when the behavior was first established.

Once you have identified the payoffs, you can create your NOW statement. To create your NOW statement, imagine that you are addressing your subconscious mind and letting it know that you are taking charge. This conversation might sound something like this: "Hey subconscious mind, I appreciate the positive intention of giving me extra sleep every morning; it's been great, but now (fill in the blank as to why you want this to change)." Or "Hey subconscious mind, I understand that by sending me into an anxiety attack every time I get in the car that you are trying to keep me safe, but now..." fill in the blank as to why you want things to change, why you are willing to give up the payoff.

*NOTE: Throughout this book, I emphasize the importance of using language that creates the imagery of what you want. It **is very** important, however, in this step, and this step only, you are identifying the problem, and it is fine to use any language that comes to mind. When you do the self-hypnosis, you will be including the solution to the problem, not only the problem itself.*

The following examples will help you get an idea about how to fill out your Personal Change Blueprint on step one, identifying your payoffs and writing your NOW statement. These are examples of how other people have answered this question.

Example 1 — Possible **payoffs/**benefits for not having financial abundance, and a NOW statement explaining why you are willing to give up those payoffs or benefits.

- **<u>Person A</u>**
- <u>Payoff for not having financial abundance</u>: I have always seen rich people as snooty and pretentious. As long as I am not rich, I will not be snooty or pretentious, and people will like me better!
- <u>My NOW statement based on this payoff</u>: Being poor has protected me from becoming snooty and pretentious, but NOW, I am certain that I will be a very kind and generous rich person. I am confident that I can do great things with my money. The fact that I am aware of the pitfalls of wealth helps to assure me that I can avoid those pitfalls.
- **<u>Person B</u>**
- <u>Payoff for not having financial abundance</u>: I have always been taught that money is the root of all evil. As long as I don't have too much money, I will avoid the evil temptations that come with financial abundance.
- <u>My NOW statement based on this payoff</u>: I grew up believing that money was the root

of all evil and rich people were not to be trusted, but NOW, I do not see how the two are connected. I am a good person as I am, and I know that having a lot of money is not going to make me evil.

- **Person C**
- <u>Payoff for not having financial abundance:</u> If I were rich, people would only love me for my money, and I would never really know if they genuinely like me or if they just think I will give them money.

- <u>My NOW statement based on this payoff:</u> Staying poor as an excuse not to trust people is only hurting me! I'm ready to move away from this belief because NOW, I trust in my ability to sense if people are sincere or not. I have no concern that I will give people money in the hopes that they will like me better. I can be responsible with money.

<u>Example 2</u> — Possible **payoffs**/benefits for not having a healthy relationship and a NOW statement explaining why you are willing to give up those payoffs or benefits.

- **Person A**
- <u>Payoff for not having a healthy relationship:</u> Having a healthy relationship with someone sounds exhausting. I would have to lose a lot

of weight to attract someone worth the trouble. I will just settle with whoever likes me the way I am, eating whatever I want.

- <u>My NOW statement based on this payoff:</u> Being alone has been a great excuse to eat whatever I want, but NOW, I am ready to take good care of my body because it is the right thing to do and, in the process, I know I can have a healthy relationship regardless of my weight.

- **Person B**

- <u>Payoff for not having a healthy relationship:</u> Having a healthy relationship is a lot of pressure. I have so many skeletons in my closet, and I do not want to take them out and show them to anyone. I would rather keep my past a secret. I hate talking about my past.

- <u>My NOW statement based on this payoff:</u> Even though talking about my past traumas is something I have avoided, I am tired of using it as an excuse to be alone. I am ready for change because, NOW, having a healthy relationship means being honest with my partner, and I am ready for a partner who will listen to me and respect me for what I have been through.

- **Person C**
- <u>Payoff for not having a healthy relationship:</u> Having a healthy relationship is too much work. I have been hurt so many times, and I am not willing to take that chance again, ever. It is just too hard!
- <u>My NOW statement based on this payoff:</u> It is true that I have been hurt several times in past relationships, but NOW, I am willing to make the necessary changes in my life to attract a healthy relationship.

Example 3 - Possible **payoffs/**benefits for not having my dream career and a NOW statement explaining why you are willing to give up those payoffs or benefits.

- **Person A**
- <u>Payoff for not having my dream career:</u> I save a lot of money because I did not have to go to school and take out any student loans.
- <u>My NOW statement based on this payoff:</u> It is true that I have saved a lot of money by not going to school, but it's not worth the level of dissatisfaction I feel going to work every day. NOW I am ready to make more money doing what I love. I'll make plenty of money to pay off my student loans.

- **Person B**
- <u>Payoff for not having my dream career:</u> I avoid rejection by not applying and interviewing for more challenging jobs.
- <u>My NOW statement based on this payoff:</u> Playing it safe has its benefits, but I know I could do better because NOW I'm ready to make more money and feel the satisfaction of doing meaningful work.
- **Person C**
- <u>Payoff for not having my dream career:</u> My current job is easy, and I do not have to risk having a job that makes me work nights.
- <u>My NOW statement based on this payoff:</u> I have the easy way out, but I'm not a teenager anymore, and NOW I'm ready to step up to the plate and meet my potential. I know I can do better—no more excuses.

Hopefully, the examples have helped you identify some of the possible payoffs and/or benefits that could be gained because of the negative or unwanted aspects in those particular areas of life. If you cannot come up with any payoffs for your situation, think back to when the situation first occurred. It might be twenty or thirty years ago. Sometimes the payoff resides in the original creation of the unwanted event. For example, if you have poor sleep habits now, think back to when it started. Your current poor sleep habits might have been helpful to you if they started when you brought your first baby home or when you were in college and had to study all night. For more help in fleshing out the payoffs and benefits from your specific situation, join our Facebook group. For details https://debbietaylor-author.com/social-media-links/loa-pcb-facebook-group/.

In Chapter Five, you will add to your Personal Change Blueprint by identifying the exact outcome you want to manifest. It seems like a simple task, but as you will learn, it is not always as easy as it seems.

"Envision the future you desire. Create the life of your dreams. See it, feel it, believe it."
Jack Canfield

Chapter Five

Step Two – Crafting Your Outcome for Exactly What You Want

This is your outcome. Sounds easy enough, yes? In step two of creating your Personal Change Blueprint, you will identify exactly what you want. Notice your thoughts when you first contemplate this idea. Did you think of what you do not want? For example, did you think, "I know absolutely what I want; I want to stop worrying about money?" Or "I don't want another dysfunctional relationship?" Or "I don't want to do this boring job for the rest of my life?"

I get it. I know what you really want even when you tell me what you don't want but think about the imagery your subconscious mind creates when you dwell on what you don't want. Remember, your subconscious mind emits the frequency of whatever you are focused on. It does not have the ability to read between the lines or interpret what you really mean.

For example, you may think you want to lose weight. But what you want is to create a lifestyle where you enjoy eating healthy foods in the right amounts at the right time, which allows your body to maintain a healthy weight. You may think you want gobs of money, when in fact, what you really want is the security of financial independence and the freedom to come and go as you please.

It may sound like I am splitting hairs here, but I want you to learn how to fine-tune your desires right down to the last detail. Sometimes it is easier to talk about the *reasons* we want a certain outcome than identifying the *actual* outcome. You want to tell the universe, through your subconscious mind, what you want to manifest. You are much more than one simple wish to quit smoking, lose weight, or get rich.

When you are writing your outcome, it is of paramount importance that you do not include any difficulties with your outcome. For example, you would not want to say, "I find it easy to eat healthy food all day unless there is a party at work, and someone brings cake." Or, "I love making a ton of money even though the IRS is going to take half of it." Or, "I look forward to attracting my perfect mate, as long as he doesn't have any kids." Get the point?

Here are some additional examples of possible outcomes based on the manifestation of financial abundance, manifesting a healthy relationship, or getting your dream career. Do not worry about the supporting details. We will address those in the following steps.

Example 1- Possible **outcomes** based on the desire to manifest financial abundance.

- I find it easy to make more than enough money to pay my bills each month.
- Money just comes to me effortlessly.
- I have the freedom to buy whatever I want at the store every week.
- I am out of debt and will remain so for the rest of my life.

Example 2 – Possible **outcomes** based on my desire to manifest a healthy relationship.

- I am confident and settled into the reality of a healthy adult relationship.
- The relationship I have with my partner is strong, healthy, and solid.
- I have a healthy relationship with an honest, trustworthy, loving partner.
- I have a healthy relationship with someone who shares my values and beliefs.

Example 3- Possible **outcomes** based on my desire to manifest my dream career.

- I have a career that reflects my intellectual abilities.
- I have a job that allows me to work part-time and I am well paid for my contribution.
- I wake up every morning looking forward to going to work each day.
- My job is so much fun, and I feel like I get paid for playing all day!

Craft your outcome carefully. Try to write it in one sentence and look at it as if it was your Personal Change Blueprint title. This outcome is the main idea of your mind movie.

As you continue working your way through each of the eight steps of your Personal Change Blueprint, remember to come back to this step each time and work your way through the subsequent steps, reviewing the answers you write as you add to the blueprint with each step. You are building and reinforcing the mind movie of what you want and letting the universe know what menu item you expect next.

The Story of Julie

A few years back, I worked with a woman whom we'll name Julie. She wanted me to help her stop ruminating about how much her husband and sister-in-law irritated her. She and her husband had moved into her sister-in-law's house a few years earlier to save money while getting their businesses up and running. Unfortunately, Julie's internal dialog was in a negative feedback loop, and all she could think of all day was how annoying they both were. Julie was quite well-versed in how the Law of Attraction worked, and she knew if she did not stop the negative rumination, it would only worsen.

It did not take long to decipher that what Julie wanted was for her and her husband was to purchase their own home and move out of her sister-in-law's house. The cost of buying a home was so far out of reach for Julie and her husband that she hadn't even considered that a possibility. She had just started a jewelry-making business, her dream career, after working in a completely unrelated industry for several years. Her income was very inconsistent and not nearly enough to purchase a home.

After turning down the volume on Julie's negative ruminations about her husband and her sister-in-law, Julie and I started crafting her Personal Change Blueprint with the focus on getting her and her husband into a home of their own. We did not include any details about how this would happen; we just focused on fleshing out her Personal Change Blueprint. Julie's outcome changed from wanting to stop complaining about her husband and sister-in-law to focusing on getting her into the right mindset about buying their own house. We didn't spend any time trying to figure out how to make this happen, we just created a Personal Change Blueprint based on what Julie really wanted, and that was to have her own home.

This is the beauty of the Law of Attraction. You do not have to figure out the how-to of manifesting what you want. You just focus on what you want.

Focusing on the how-to is a great way to sabotage your manifestation because then you start worrying about roadblocks and obstacles standing between where you are and where you want to be. Trying to figure out how to get what you want often leads to focusing on its absence. It is like ordering off the menu at a restaurant. You just order what you want. What goes on behind closed doors in the kitchen is of no concern to you. You do not worry about where they got the vegetables you just ordered, whether the pan is clean enough to cook in, or if the cook knows how to make mashed potatoes. You just order what you want and then enjoy yourself, knowing that somehow, someway, someone is magically putting that meal together for you, just the way you asked. Law of Attraction is like that.

Let's get back to Julie's story. It was not long after Julie and I finished working together when she called to tell me to say that on a whim, she had decided to check the job boards at the firm she used to work for. They had an opening that was perfect for her. She applied and was offered a job paying substantially more than she had ever made. While she loved the idea of running her own jewelry-making business, the truth was, it was not turning out to be the dream career she thought it would be. She happily went back to her former career. She called to tell me that she and her husband had just closed on their very own house. She couldn't have been happier.

Julie and I could have stayed focused on the thought habit of thinking negatively about her husband and sister-in-law. It turns out that the thought habit she had was not the problem but a symptom of the real problem. Take this into consideration as you craft the outcome statement on your Personal Change Blueprint.

In the next chapter, you will learn about step three in creating your Personal Change Blueprint. Step three is all about brainstorming the changes you will notice because you have manifested your desired outcome. You will be citing the evidence of your Law of Attraction mastery.

"Whatever you hold in your mind on a consistent basis is exactly what you will experience in your life."
Tony Robbins

Chapter Six

Step Three - Your Evidence

From the perspective of already having manifested your desire in step two, your outcome, what kind of change does that make in your daily routine? What do you notice? What *evidence* shows that you have accomplished your outcome, that it has simply become the new norm for you? What is different now? There will be a lot of variety in this answer.

As with each of the following questions on your Personal Change Blueprint, always start by reviewing the answers to the previous questions starting with step two, the outcome. Review it and say it back to yourself as if you were telling a story; add details, embellish it, all the while making certain to use language that creates the imagery of what you desire. When you get to step four, you will review and tell the story you have written, starting with steps two and three. When you get to step five, you will review and tell the story you have written, going over the answers to steps two, three, and four, and so on for the rest of the Personal Change Blueprint.

Here are some examples for step three based on the evidence you might notice because you manifested financial abundance, a healthy relationship, or your dream career.

Example 1 — **Evidence** that I have manifested the financial abundance I desire:

- I sleep better at night knowing that there is plenty of money to pay off my debts now and always.
- My partner and I enjoy going out to dinner anytime we feel like it, and we are free to order whatever we want every time.
- When I leave a tip, I do so freely and generously.

- I look around my house, and if I see furniture that needs to be replaced, I notice it with a sense of joy and anticipation of the fun that comes with shopping for new furniture!
- I love knowing that if my kids run into financial troubles, I have the resources to help them.
- Now when I surf the Internet looking at exotic vacation places, it is not just daydreaming. I am planning a vacation; there are no limits to where I can go!

Example 2 — **Evidence** that I have manifested a fantastic healthy relationship:

- I feel valued as a person.
- When I am with my partner, I am free to express my thoughts and feelings, knowing that I am heard and my opinions count.
- I always feel good about how I look when I leave the house because I dress to please myself, no one else. My partner loves me no matter how I look.
- Intimacy has never been more fun! Everything just clicks; we are in sync with each other's likes and dislikes, yet we remain individually true to ourselves.

- We like each other's friends, and there is a high level of mutual respect. There are no red flags, only green ones.
- I feel content, present with what is, free from any compulsion to run away in fear or insisting on a premature commitment.

Example 3 — **Evidence** that I have manifested my dream career.

- At night when I get in bed to go to sleep, I drift off to sleep with a smile on my face, excited about what the morning will bring.
- I love waking up knowing that I get to go to a job where my views are respected, I am treated as a professional, and I am well paid for the work I do.
- I enjoy the people I work with, and it just feels right when I am at work. I am good at what I do.
- People want to hear what I have to say, and my confidence is going through the roof! I feel better about myself all around because I was hired for this job.
- I love going to work in the morning, and when it is time to go home, it feels like it has only been a few hours since I got there!

- There is plenty of room for growth in this organization, and I am grateful every day for this opportunity.

The Story of Anna

Anna was single, retired, but still young and energetic enough to work. She needed to work, but what she wanted most was to run her own business. Her energy—her vibrational frequency—was split.

On the one hand, she wanted and needed to find a job that would pay her bills, and on the other hand, she wanted enough capital to get her business up and running, knowing that most home businesses do not show a profit for several years. She spent a lot of time ruminating on the idea that she did not have enough money to pay for the certification class she needed to open her own business. Running her own business felt like a pipe dream. She set the dream aside and decided to go back to school to get yet another degree so she could get a good-paying job. By going back to school, she would at least have financial aid money to help pay the bills. She would deal with the student debt later.

Anna's understanding of the Law of Attraction was minimal at best. She was in survival mode and just wanted enough financial security to take her mind off the ever-growing possibility of losing everything and having to file bankruptcy. She put the dream of running her own business on the back burner and settled into the life of a full-time student living off student loans again. And then a strange thing happened.

Anna got an email notification about a job that had become available in her area. Previously, she had registered with the state employment department but had never been contacted until this moment. She called the number on the notice and scheduled an interview for a teaching position that she was overqualified for, but it was a job.

Anna was offered and accepted the job. The pay was just barely enough to keep her head above water, and then it dawned on her. Now that she was making a little extra money, she would have just enough extra student loan money to pay for the certification course she needed to open her own business. Not only did Anna's new job give her the financial edge she needed to get the appropriate certification, but she was off work each day at three o'clock in the afternoon. This schedule gave her three to four hours each day to work at the business she was opening without the pressure of *needing* to make a certain amount of money to keep the business open.

Anna's new job paid her just enough money to keep the collection agencies off her back, which is what she asked for, but it did not pay her enough to make it hard to leave when the time came. Anna worked at both jobs, the teaching job and growing her own business, for three years until she felt confident enough to quit the teaching job and make her living by running her own business.

This story illustrates the importance of focusing on what you want and letting the powers that be figure out the "how-to" of the manifestation. Anna got everything she wanted, but she could never have imagined it all coming together the way it did. Focus on how it feels to have what you want without fussing over the "how-to" of it. You just have to let the details work themselves out and trust that the chef in the kitchen knows what he's doing.

In the next chapter, you will start tapping into your imagination even more than you already have. As you review your Personal Change Blueprint up to this point, you will start to develop some imagery to go along with it. Chapter Six is all about documenting that imagery.

"Thoughts become things. If you see it in your mind, you will hold it in your hand."
Bob Proctor

Chapter Seven
Step Four – Imagery Associated with Your Manifestation

You may notice that steps four, five, and six are quite similar. The goal with these steps is to connect you with your sensory experience of living *as if* you had accomplished your outcome. The answers to the questions in these steps can be literal or figurative. In other words, when asked what your manifestation looks like if you see rainbows and butterflies, then rainbows and butterflies it is.

Before you start writing answers to this step, go back to your outcome and review it. Tell yourself the story of your manifestation using the answers you have written so far. Feel free to embellish, allowing the energy to flow. Remember to keep your answers free from difficulties and use language to create the imagery of what you want to manifest. It is normal and perfectly acceptable to repeat information from any of the other steps. Here are some examples to clarify step four and what *images* might come to mind if you were to manifest financial abundance, a healthy relationship, or your dream career.

Example 1 — Because I have manifested financial abundance in my life, **I can see:**

- I see myself standing on the bow of a yacht with the wind in my hair, and I am free!
- I see myself living in a beautiful house, tastefully decorated, and feeling completely at home.
- I see myself having all the time in the world to work on my art projects, dig in the garden, and volunteer at the local pet shelter down the street.
- I see myself as happy, content, complete. And the people around me are happy as well. I look healthy and fit because I take

good care of my body, I eat right, and I have a personal trainer come to the house on a regular basis.

- I see lots of family parties at my house, and everyone is having a good time! My face is relaxed, at ease. I am present.

Example 2 — Because I have manifested a healthy relationship in my life, **I can see:**

- I see myself waking up every morning happy to see the person next to me!
- I see a permanent grin on my face because I have arrived where I want to be in a relationship.
- I see that my partner and I have so much in common, and yet we both maintain our individuality.
- The sex is great!
- We do everything together. I see us sharing the daily tasks of cooking, sitting down for dinner, walking our dogs, and enjoying the ending of a perfect day, every day.
- I see that my partner is the perfect match for what I want in life, and I see harmony in my home. My heart is full!

<u>Example 3</u> — Because I have manifested my dream career, **I can see**

- I see myself waking up in the morning fully rested and excited to get up and get the day going.
- I see myself doing meaningful work every day, and I can see myself at work staying on task all day, every day.
- I see myself participating in group projects and running some of them.
- I see that people at work like me and want to hear what I have to say.
- I see myself expressing my views with confidence because I am good at what I do.
- I see my bank account growing and growing because I am well-compensated for doing work that I love.
- I see myself driving to work every day with a huge smile on my face!

If you are not an especially visual person, you may not have a lot to write for this step. No worries - just jot down whatever comes to mind. This information is all about you and is very personal. You do not have to share this with anyone unless you choose to. You may also find that you are a *very* visual person and can fill page after page with images that come to mind when you think of what this accomplishment looks like. Make it yours. The sky is the limit!

The Story of Lisa

Lisa grew up in the city but was a country girl at heart. She longed for a home in the country. In her mind's eye, she could see this little farmhouse out in the middle of nowhere, surrounded by a white picket fence. She loved the idea of living where there were no neighbors, just space. In her imagination, she would always see this house as if she were hovering above it like an angel.

Lisa did not know about the Law of Attraction. She simply lived day to day below the veil of consciousness like almost everyone else on the planet. She would get up in the morning, feed her kids, drop them off at school, and head to work. Day after day, Lisa carried on, never realizing that she had the power within herself to improve her daily life experience. She was not miserable, but she was not especially happy either.

Several years later, Lisa began exploring various spiritual teachings and ran across the teachings of Esther Hicks. She learned about the Law of Attraction and liked the idea of manifesting a new house, a fancy car, and a lot of money, but soon realized that just wishing for those things did not make them so. Lisa believed it was possible to manifest a better life, but she had no idea how to make it happen, and so she carried on with the status quo.

Many things changed in Lisa's life over the years, but one thing remained, and that was the dream of living in that little farmhouse out in the middle of nowhere—the house with the white picket fence. She would daydream about it regularly, especially at night before she drifted off to sleep.

Lisa graduated from college, raised her kids, and made the decision to move to another state. She settled in a very remote town where she was hired to teach elementary school. She was finally out of the city and had access to the peaceful life she had always imagined for herself. The rivers and mountains she loved to spend time in were just a short drive away.

Over time, she moved from one home to another within the same small town—a town so small that you could see the whole of it from a single aerial photograph. It just so happened that the local diner had a collection of aerial photographs of the town and all the surrounding ranchlands, showing the changes from years ago up to the present time.

Lisa enjoyed looking at the pictures, comparing certain places from what they looked like years ago to what they looked like today. One day while looking at the photographs, she recognized the little house she was living in. She could see it all from the aerial perspective, and that is when it hit her. Her dream, her fantasy house, was right there in front of her. She was living in a little farmhouse with a picket fence around it, out in the middle of ranchland. It was just as she had always seen in her mind, and yet she had never put two and two together until now. All those years of dreaming and fantasizing about living in that little house had finally come to fruition.

Lisa's story is an important lesson for all of us. Be aware of what you dream about and have faith that your dreams can come true. Keep your dreams alive and visit them often. Take a look at your current situation and ask yourself, "How did I dream this into being?" If you are not happy with your current manifestation, dream a new one into being.

In the next chapter, you will learn how to identify specific sounds associated with the manifestation of your outcome. This detail is overlooked by many people. Sounds are an important part of our daily life experience. What sounds will you notice?

"Love what you want. Believe wholeheartedly what you want, imagine that you're already having it. You will DEFINITELY get it. This is how it works!"
Aanoor Pradeep

Chapter Eight
Step Five - Sounds Associated with Your Manifestation

Are you beginning to see how your mind movie is coming together? You have identified what you want, and you have described the changes happening in your life because you have manifested what you want. You know now what images come to mind when you think about this manifestation, and in step five, you will identify the sounds associated with this manifestation. Review your story again, beginning with the outcome. Take your time and let the imagery and the details expand.

If you are an auditory learner, this step will be easy for you, and you have probably already started writing. If you are not an auditory learner, you will appreciate that when I talk about associated sounds related to your manifestation, they can fall into any or all of the following three areas:

1. Associated sounds can include your internal dialogue, the thoughts in your mind. What is that voice in your head saying about accomplishing this outcome?
2. Associated sounds can include comments from other people. Will your friends, family members, coworkers, or even strangers have anything to say about this manifestation? What will they say?
3. Associated sounds can include the "absence" of a sound. This might be the absence of negative rumination or worry about things. The absence of the sound of your partner complaining about your smoking habit. The absence of the sound of you gasping for air when you walk up the stairs. The sound of stillness, the sound of peace, and metaphorically, the sound of contentment might be part of what you hear.

Write down as much as you can, remembering that when you are reviewing this information later, or when you are in self-hypnosis, you are free to add any additional relevant details that come to mind at that point.

The following examples will help you understand more about **associated sounds** related to the manifestation of financial abundance, a healthy relationship, or a dream career.

Example 1- The **sounds associated** with the manifestation of financial abundance may include:

- The sound of my keyboard as I type in my bank account number to check my balance as it grows and grows!
- I hear myself talking with my financial manager as they advise me about investments.
- I hear the voice in my head screaming with joy about all the opportunities available to me now that I have unlimited funds.
- I hear my spouse telling me how grateful he/she is for our financial abundance.
- I hear the sound of laughter coming from my kids while we're on vacation, and they are having the time of their lives.

- I hear the absence of a noisy car engine because my new Tesla is dead quiet.

Example 2- The **sounds associated** with the manifestation of a healthy relationship may include:

- The sounds of pleasure, the moaning, and groaning of a great sex life!
- I hear the voice in my head having great conversations with my partner about our dinner plans or our vacation plans while I am away during the day.
- I hear the sweetness of my partner's voice telling me that I am loved and appreciated.
- I notice the clear absence of a raised voice or an angry exchange.
- I hear stillness in my heart.

Example 3- The **sounds associated** with the manifestation of my dream career may include:

- The sound of my voice in a team meeting interacting and contributing value to the project.
- The confidence in my voice while I consult with my manager about any part of my job. I hear kindness coming from my coworkers.

- My coworkers' voices are respectful toward me, and they ask questions that I confidently answer.
- The voice in my head is all positive.
- I constantly hear my internal voice expressing joy and gratitude for landing this job.
- I hear myself proudly telling people what kind of work I do.
- There is a clear absence of any negative thoughts, worries, or ruminations about needing a different job. I hear my body and mind in sync with each other.
- I hear myself speaking with confidence and clearly articulating my ideas at work.

You may be surprised at how many sounds are associated with the manifestation you are working on. If you are bothered by the habit of negative thoughts, remember, they are just thought *habits*. See yourself with a magical remote control, and anytime you become aware that your brain is thinking thoughts you do not want to think, imagine picking up that remote and either changing the channel, turning off the thoughts, or directing your attention to something more pleasing. Make a deal with yourself right here and now to never finish a thought about something you do not want to experience.

The Story of Dana

Dana and I have had many conversations about the Law of Attraction and how to harness the power of the subconscious mind. True to the scientist she is, Dana likes to put things to the test to see how they hold up under scrutiny. She wanted to believe in the Law of Attraction but had difficulty telling the difference between an intentional manifestation and a coincidence.

Dana readily accepted a challenge I gave her. I asked her to think of something she would like to manifest, something simple but unique and out of the ordinary. She was to spend a few minutes imagining this object in the privacy of her own mind before going to sleep, just for one night. I told her to imagine the object as if it were suspended in space, to let it turn slowly so she could get a good look at every angle. Then she was to imagine her hand reaching out and holding or touching the object so she could get a good idea of its relative size. Her assignment was to do this just once, for five minutes.

She chose to focus on something simple yet unique to test the Law of Attraction to see if she could manifest an object. She chose to focus on a kewpie doll. A kewpie doll was commonly given as a prize at carnivals and amusement parks in the fifties and sixties. It is a little doll with rosy cheeks and a tuft of curly hair on its head. A unique object that you do not see every day.

Dana did as instructed and visualized the kewpie doll in the privacy of her mind for five minutes one night before sleep. A few days later, she cut through an antique store on her way back to her car from a farmer's market. She was making her way to the exit when she looked up, and there it was—her kewpie doll! She was amazed for about ten seconds and then discounted the whole thing because an antique store is exactly where you would expect to find a kewpie doll. She was not convinced. Not yet.

I asked her to pick another out-of-the-ordinary object and to follow the same process. This time she chose a whiffle ball. A whiffle ball is a white, hollow plastic ball with dime-size holes cut into its surface all around. A few days later, Dana was at an amusement park with her family. They were walking around deciding which ride to get on next when she walked past a game with a giant tub of water that just happened to be full of whiffle balls. Again, she was amazed for about ten seconds and then discounted the whole thing because an amusement park is exactly where you would expect to find a whiffle ball.

One more time. I encouraged Dana to come up with another object that she was unlikely to run across anywhere in her travels. She chose a skeleton key. Neither of us could imagine any scenario where she would inadvertently run across a skeleton key. She followed the same process as before, imagining every detail of her skeleton key from top to bottom.

At this point, Dana was losing interest in testing the theory about the Law of Attraction and simply carried on with her regular routine. The following day, she opened her Facebook feed as usual and was scrolling when she came upon a post from one of her friends who was excitedly showing off her new tattoo on the inside of her right forearm. There it was, in living color, a beautiful tattoo of a skeleton key. Dana gasped and called me immediately. This time she was amazed for more than ten seconds. She was a believer!

This is a fun exercise anyone can do. Think of an object you are unlikely to run across in the ordinary course of your day. Right before you drift off to sleep, spend five minutes imagining your object. See it as if it were suspended in space and let it rotate slowly in front of you so you can see every detail, every angle. Imagine yourself reaching out and holding or touching the object to give yourself an idea of its relative size, and then don't give it another thought. I think you will be pleasantly surprised at your ability to manifest in such a short time.

In the next chapter, you will be learning how to answer the question about feelings in step six. This includes physical and emotional feelings. You are doing an excellent job at creating new neural pathways in your brain, and you are doing an excellent job at training your subconscious mind to emit the same vibration as your conscious mind. Once you begin doing this while in the state of hypnosis, you will start to notice tangible evidence of your progress. Keep up the good work.

"Whatever you're thinking about is literally like planning a future event. When you're worrying, you are planning. When you're appreciating, you are planning ... What are you planning?"
Thoughtnova.com

Chapter Nine
Step Six - Physical and
Emotional Feelings

When I work with clients one on one, this step consistently gets the most answers. You may have noticed in previous steps that when you asked yourself about imagery or sounds, you naturally answered with words describing what it felt like instead of, or in addition to, what it looked or sounded like.

In this step, like the previous steps, review your answers, starting with the outcome. Read them to yourself out loud as if you were telling a grand story. Feel free to add details as they come to you. As you repeat your story over and over, you are accomplishing three things: first, you are creating new neural pathways in your brain, which will result in new habits of thought, new physical habits, rituals, and routines; second, you are modifying the vibrational frequency being sent out by the subconscious part of your mind in regard to this subject; and third, you are telling the Universe what you want, what it looks like, what it sounds like, what it feels like, and more. This is how you master the Law of Attraction by aligning the frequency of the subconscious mind with the frequency of the conscious mind.

Here are some examples to help you understand more about how to describe what it **feels** like, **physically and/or emotionally**, to manifest financial abundance, a healthy relationship, or your dream career.

Example 1- The **feelings, physical and/or emotional**, associated with the manifestation of financial abundance might include:

- The feeling of relief. I feel a huge relief like a giant weight has been taken off my shoulders.
- I feel light and airy like I could fly to the moon, and excited to know that I can pay off my debt, all of it.
- I feel proud to know that I can support my family in style and move us into a house with room for everyone.
- I also feel very happy to know that I can donate to worthy charities and help others less fortunate.

Example 2 - The **feelings, physical and/or emotional** associated with the manifestation of a healthy relationship might include:

- The feeling of being in love, but a more authentic mature feeling of love.
- I feel content because I know my partner is on the same page as me.
- I am happy to have a life partner with the same values as mine.
- I feel giddy sometimes, like a schoolgirl, but this is real, not just a crush.
- The reality of this relationship washes over me sometimes with such sweetness!
- I am grateful beyond description, and my heart is bursting with love.

- I feel vibrant, alive, alert like I am going to burst wide open!

Example 3 - The **feelings, physical and/or emotional** associated with the manifestation of finding your dream career might include:

- The feeling of being proud! I love my work, and it feels amazing to know that I am contributing to the world by doing meaningful work every day.
- I look forward to getting up in the morning, every morning, even on Monday mornings!
- I have fun interacting with my coworkers. They have accepted me as one of the gang, and it feels good to be respected and to have other professionals seek my opinion.
- I feel like I am living up to my potential.
- I feel like a grown-up, able to carry on and take care of my family like a truly responsible adult.

The information you put down on this step of your Personal Change Blueprint can be extensive. That is okay. Getting in touch with your feelings sends out a powerful vibrational frequency. When it comes to making the Law of Attraction work, I always say, "You can say all the pretty words you want, but if you are not feeling those words, they won't do you any good. Your frequency is emitting what you feel more than what you say."

The Story of Marlene

Marlene came to me to get help with weight loss. She was not obese but wanted to lose about forty pounds. She had a happy marriage, a job she loved, and a house full of teenagers, including a teenage foreign exchange student. She loved cooking for everyone. Her kitchen was filled with all the kinds of foods you would expect to see in a house full of teens: chips, sodas, doughnuts, pizza, ice cream, and more.

Marlene used to be a runner, and she felt that if she could change her eating habits and start running again, she would be able to kick start her "old" self into being once again.

We worked on her Personal Change Blueprint based on the outcome of weight loss. The interesting thing about the Personal Change Blueprint is that it takes you far beyond the simple one-line description of what you want. Marlene's answers to each of the steps helped her identify a new way of living that went far beyond the manifestation of weight loss.

About one year after I had worked with Marlene, she sent me an email thanking me for the work we did together. Here is a copy of her email to me:

Dear Debbie,

I've been wanting to write you for a while now to let you know how much I appreciate all the help you gave me with hypnosis. If you remember, I came in for weight loss. Well, I lost the weight, but I got so much more out of our work together than just losing weight! Losing the weight turned out to be quite easy, but the best part is that I found myself again. I didn't realize how much being "lost" was interfering with my health until you helped me figure out what it would feel like to be back in my own skin again. You helped me tap into my internal resources at a depth I didn't know existed. I feel as though a fog has been lifted from my mind, and I can see clearly again.

I am grateful to you for your help. Thank you for guiding me through this process.

Respectfully, Marlene

As you continue this process, you will be awakening thoughts and feeling inside that have been dormant for a long time. Welcome those feelings, embrace the new way of seeing, hearing, and feeling how you want your life to be. Develop the habit of opening up to the reality that you can manifest the kind of life you want for yourself in the here and now.

In the next chapter, you are going to change gears just a bit. In step seven, you will go over all your answers and then take some time to contemplate what this change does for you. The work you are doing will have far-reaching consequences, not just for you but for your whole family and possibly your friends. This is the time to open up to the value of what you are doing.

*"Imagination is everything; it is the preview
of life's coming attractions."*
Albert Einstein

Chapter Ten

Step Seven - What Does Change
Do for You?

This is a good time to step back and take a wide-angle look at this mind movie you have created for yourself. You have invested a lot of energy into figuring out what the payoffs are, or were, for having this unwanted habit or situation. You evaluated that payoff and agreed that you were willing to give up any and all benefits coming from it in exchange for what you truly want. You identified what you want clearly and concisely, in the form of an outcome. Once you identified your outcome, you identified the changes that would occur because you had accomplished your outcome. You listed the evidence proving to yourself that change had indeed occurred. You noticed and documented what those changes look like, sound like, and feel like.

Here in step seven, I want you to take it all in. Imagine yourself a year down the road, or five years down the road, and tell me, "What does having this change do for you?"

In other words, *why is this so important? What does it mean in the big scheme of things?* I want you to take a moment and understand at a deep level why this outcome is so important. As always, I have examples below to help you understand more about how you might answer this question based on the manifestation of financial abundance, a healthy relationship, or your dream career.

Example 1- **What does it do for me** to have manifested financial abundance?

- Having manifested financial abundance allows me to live my life in peace and pursue other dreams and interests with emotional stability.
- Now I can focus on other aspects of life without feeling like I am in survival mode all the time. I know that if a health issue

comes up, I have the money to do all that I can to help myself.

- If my spouse or one of our kids has any accident or injury, I know I can afford the best treatment available.
- If my car breaks down, I know I have the money to fix it.
- With financial wellness in hand, I can move forward in life with grace and ease.

Example 2 - **What does it do for me** to have manifested a healthy relationship?

- Having a healthy relationship gives me an internal sense of peace, as though the quest is over, and I can settle into living life, creating a family of my own, and feeling like I have found that missing element.
- Having a healthy relationship gives me the confidence to know that because I have successfully manifested this into my life, I can manifest anything I want at any time.
- I feel like I belong to the "happy family" club now. I'm a normal human being.

Example 3 - **What does it do for me** to have manifested my dream career?

- Having manifested my dream career makes me feel fulfilled, like I am living up to my potential.
- I know I am a good role model for my kids, and the internal satisfaction I feel can only be good for my health! I feel smart and capable and worthy.
- I do not "need" other people to approve of me, but it sure feels good to know that my work is valued and that I am making a positive contribution to this world.

One of the most common answers to this question is the idea that because I have manifested this outcome, I know now that I can do anything. Sometimes it just takes one experience to crack that barrier keeping us from living our best life. I am convinced that once you start to see real-life proof that you can make the Law of Attraction work in your favor, you will be off to the races.

One of my favorite pieces of advice learned from listening to Esther Hicks speaking for Abraham is this: "There is no competition for wellness. There is enough wellness to go around for all of us!"

I think it is safe to say that the idea of wellness encompasses all aspects of our lives. It is easy in our culture to feel like we have to win all the time, be the best or the biggest or get there first. If you can remember the advice above, it will be easier for you to take things in stride. There is no hurry about any of this. There is enough wellness for all of us.

The Story of Me and My Old House

When I divorced, I was awarded the booby prize of an old house dating back to 1901. This house was built before indoor plumbing, and not too long after electricity was the norm. There was only one electrical outlet in each room. Talk about outdated wiring. This was an old home that had been added onto every twenty years since it was first built, and each addition had a downward tilt toward the side of the house it was built on. There was no foundation. It was built on a wood frame, and the bathroom, being an afterthought, was put in where the original back porch was.

This was not a "charming" turn of the century home. It was an eyesore and a money pit, and all I wanted to do was fix it up and get rid of it—quickly.

The first thing I did was to have a foundation poured underneath the house. Apparently, you cannot get a loan on a house if it does not have a foundation. My ex-husband had purchased the home for $13,000 cash ten years earlier, so the lack of foundation had not been an issue. Once the foundation was in, I noticed that whenever I would open any of the interior doors, they would scrape across the very bowed wood floor. I needed to get a contractor to take a look and tell me what could be done to fix that.

For an entire year, I called numerous contractors and left messages explaining my situation and asking them to call me back to make an appointment and give me a bid. None of them ever called me back. It became a joke with my friends, and I started saying that I needed to date a carpenter to fix the floors and replace the windows, a plumber to replace the outdated pipes in the bathroom, an electrician to rewire every room and add a few more outlets, and an all-around handyman to help clean out the attic, fix the fence, install a dishwasher, and so on. The list of men I needed to date was meant to be a joke, but it became my motto, and I would rattle off this list anytime the subject of my home renovation came up, which was quite often. Little did I know I was sending out that request into the universe.

The only part of this renovation I could do without help was the painting. So, I painted every room, ten-foot ceilings with four sections of decorative wood trim on every wall: chair rail molding, crown molding, baseboard molding, and another piece exactly twelve inches from the ceiling. And of course, all the woodwork was a different color than the walls. By the time I got ready to paint the exterior, I was exhausted.

I remember the day I was at the hardware store waiting in line to have some paint mixed for the outside of the house. There was a man in front of me buying supplies for what looked like a major project. As if someone else were speaking through me, I blurted out and asked him if he was a contractor. He was. I told him about my bowed wood floors and asked him if he thought he could fix such a thing. He offered to follow me home to look at the floors and give me a bid. I was shocked— after all this time, someone was finally going to take a look at my floors.

Here comes the amazing part. This guy not only came over to look at the floors, but he also toured the rest of the house as I explained everything that needed to be done. He saw that I was getting ready to paint the outside of the house and offered to loan me his paint sprayer, and of course, I said yes. Long story short, he became a good friend of mine and turned out to be a jack-of-all-trades. Fast forward six months, and I had new plumbing, new wiring, new windows, a flat refinished floor, an empty attic and garage, and a fixed fence, all at cost. Talk about manifesting! I never dreamed that I could find all those skills in one person, but that is exactly what I had manifested. The house looked great, and I sold it in a relatively short amount of time and made a new friend in the process.

You never know *how* your manifestations will come to you, and it is a good thing we do not have to worry about the how-to part. Nine times out of ten, your outcomes will manifest in ways that are bigger and better than anything you could ever have imagined. I know I never imagined getting my house renovated by just one person and making a new friend in the process. Keep your focus on what you want and how it feels to have it right here and now. That is how you rewire your subconscious mind, and it is the subconscious mind that is putting in your order from the Universal Menu of Manifestations.

You are finally ready for the last step of your Personal Change Blueprint! In step eight, you will fill in any missing details in various areas and then be ready to learn how to apply your Personal Change Blueprint in self-hypnosis. This truly is the secret behind *The Secret*.

*"How you vibrate is what the universe echoes
back to you in every moment."*
Panache

Chapter Eleven

Step Eight - Positive Influences

One more step to fill out in your Personal Change Blueprint, and you will be ready to learn how to do self-hypnosis—the easiest part of this entire process. There is a slight catch, though. This step has five parts to it.

Not to worry. After working your way through the previous seven steps, you will find it easy to fill in these last details. In fact, you may find that the answers to the questions in this step have already been addressed in some of the previous steps. If that is the case, feel free to write those answers again or add entirely new ideas. Also, if nothing comes to mind in any part of this section, that is okay too. The idea here is to think about the kind of **positive influences** you will notice in each of the following categories: relationships, career/ finances, health, self-esteem, and spirituality because you have manifested financial abundance, a healthy relationship, or your dream career.

Category 1- **Relationships**

Example 1 - **Positive influence on relationships** because I have manifested financial abundance.

- I feel more comfortable accepting invitations from friends who travel a lot because I can easily afford to join them.
- My partner and I are getting along better because I have a lot less stress in my life.
- I enjoy contributing to charitable causes, and I am just easier to get along with overall.

Example 2- **Positive influence on relationships** because I have manifested a healthy relationship.

- My friends and extended family members are very happy for me. They can see that I feel happy, content and take better care of myself, and they feel relieved.

- My partner and I are both incredibly happy to be in a mature, adult, functional relationship, and we are both kinder to everyone because we feel better about ourselves.

Example 3- **Positive influence on relationships** because I have manifested the ideal career for me.

- Because I feel more confident about myself, I am more at ease around my friends, family, and people at work.
- My stress levels are down because I enjoy the work I do, and with less stress, I experience more presence, compassion, and joy overall. This allows me to be more authentic in relationships.
- The people in my environment can sense my happiness, and somehow it makes them feel better to be around me because of it.

Category 2- **Career/Finances** (if you are a student, replace career with education.)

Example 1- **Positive influence on my career/ finances** because I have manifested financial abundance.

- I enjoy the work and enjoy knowing that I am well paid.

- Because money is no object, I can focus on work tasks and feel good about working overtime when I need to.
- I do a better job at work each day because I am free from the frustration of wishing I had a better job.
- I look great because I can afford to wear nice, quality suits, and I feel more professional.
- People respect me more, and I feel like I am giving quality work every day.

Example 2- **Positive influence on my career/ finances** because I have manifested a healthy relationship.

- Having a healthy relationship has decreased my stress levels, and that shows up in the quality of work I do every day.
- I am happy knowing that there are no empty spots in my life.
- My partner and I enjoy socializing with some of my workmates on occasion.
- My happiness has been a good influence on my overall attitude at work.

Example 3- **Positive influence on career/ finances** because I have manifested my dream career.

- The search is over, I have found the career that feeds my soul, and it is easy to give 100% every single day.
- Having manifested this career makes it fun to go to work every day.
- My contribution to various projects at work is going to land me a promotion very soon, and I am up to the task.

Category 3- **Health**:

Example 1- **Positive influence on my health** because I have manifested financial abundance.

- My health is better because I can afford a gym membership and some exercise equipment at home as well.
- I buy organic food only and have no desire to drown my frustrations in alcohol. Having financial well-being has relieved the stress that used to keep me up at night.
- I sleep all through the night, uninterrupted. I look better, and I feel better.

Example 2- **Positive influence on my health** because I have manifested a healthy relationship.

- Having a healthy relationship has made it so easy to eat right and take better care of myself.

- My partner and I love to go running together and cook healthy meals together.
- We have a great sex life and wake up happy every morning.
- We both want to live a long and healthy life together, and we know we can make that happen.

Example 3- **Positive influence on health** because I have manifested the ideal career for me.

- I love my job so much, and that is having a significant influence on my physical and emotional health.
- My stress levels are so much less than they used to be, and I enjoy taking healthy lunches and snacks to work each day because it is the right thing to do.
- My job energizes me, and I find myself compelled to work out regularly.
- I sleep so well, waking up each morning well-rested, satisfied, and eager for the day because every day is another day that I get to go to work doing what I love and I am well paid for it!

Category 4- **Self-esteem**

Example 1- **Positive influence on my self-esteem** because I have manifested financial abundance.

- I am proud of the fact that I can provide for myself and my family the way I do.
- It is wonderful to buy new cars that are attractive, safe, and environmentally friendly without regard to cost.
- I feel good about the fact that I did not let old programming defeat me, causing me to live the same life my parents lived.
- I know it is just money, but it is a symbol to me, a symbol that I have what it takes to live up to my potential.

Example 2- **Positive influence on my self-esteem** because I have manifested a healthy relationship.

- I feel better about the quality people I draw into my life.
- I have proven to myself that I can attract a mature functional adult as a partner.
- It makes me feel so good about myself, and I no longer feel trapped by old programs inherited from my past.
- I have a partner that treats me with respect, which makes me feel so much better about myself!

Example 3- **Positive influence on my self-esteem** because I have manifested my dream career.

- I did it! I earned this job with hard work and perseverance.
- I feel validated to have this job!
- No one handed this to me; I qualified for this job, I interviewed for this job, and I was chosen over some other very qualified individuals because I am all that!
- I do not mean to sound arrogant, but this makes me feel so good.
- This is a validation that my intelligence is real and that I know what I am doing.

Category 5- **Spirituality** (if you do not have a spiritual practice that is an integral part of your life, feel free to leave this section blank.)

Example 1- **Positive influence on my spiritual practice** because I have manifested financial abundance.

- I love going to retreats, but I have never been able to afford them until now. Not only can I go to the retreats, but I can also afford to take time off work to do so.
- I could take a year off work and spend time doing missionary work if I wanted to.

- I will contribute financially to some of the programs my church has to help those less fortunate.
- My relationship with source has always been strong, and now there are no distractions.
- I can continue to study and join any groups I want to further my understanding of spirituality.

Example 2- **Positive influence on my spiritual practice** because I have manifested a healthy relationship.

- My partner and I enjoy discussing spiritual ideas and philosophies.
- We each have different perspectives, and as we share our ideas with each other, we are both growing and expanding beyond anything we have known before.
- Our spiritual practice is important to each of us. I am grateful that we can allow each other to have their own beliefs and feel comfortable sharing those ideas.

Example 3- **Positive influence on my spiritual practice** because I have manifested my dream career.

- My spiritual practice makes it easy for me to be present with people at work, making me a better employee.
- Because of my spiritual practice and beliefs, I find it easy to accept people for who they are and how they see the world.
- Working with other people each day allows me to practice presence and honor my belief systems.
- This job has strengthened my spiritual practice by eliminating the old negative thought patterns of wishing I was somewhere else every day.

Congratulations, you did it! You finished your Personal Change Blueprint!

You may not know it, but you have already started to rewire your brain just by creating your Personal Change Blueprint. I have always thought that the hypnosis part of this process is just the icing on the cake. The process you have just completed, filling out the eight-step Personal Change Blueprint, has already begun to make changes in your brain and the frequency your subconscious mind is sending out. You may already be seeing some evidence of your manifestation.

The Story of Carol

Carol was a people pleaser. She thought if she was nice enough and if she loved him enough, her partner would start treating her with more kindness and respect. For eight years, Carol walked on eggshells and tried to keep the peace at home. She grew up in a codependent household with a narcissistic father, and every relationship she had ever been in was based on this model. It took a while, but Carol finally started to see the patterns in her failed relationships and realized that *she* was the common denominator.

Carol had wanted to leave the relationship she was in for a long time, but she and her partner's finances were so intertwined that she could not imagine having enough money to support herself if she left. There was simply no way out, and so she stayed, year after year after year.

After eight years, things at home came to a head. Carol finally had enough of the screaming and yelling, enough of the criticism and name-calling, enough of ducking to avoid the flying objects thrown in her direction. Something snapped inside, and she made up her mind late one night that when the lease was up on the house she and her partner had just moved into, she would move. Carol had come to this conclusion before but had always backtracked because there was never the possibility of supporting herself financially. She had been stuck.

But it was different this time. Carol did not even give the concern of how she would support herself financially a second thought. There was absolutely no worry in her mind at all. All she knew was that she had to leave and that this time, she would.

Carol spent time daydreaming, fantasizing about the relief of being out of that house and away from the destructive environment she had lived in for eight years. She never gave a thought to where she would live or how she would afford it. She was content to immerse herself in the absolute joy of freedom from the emotional pain and fear of staying.

Carol's daughter and her family were just five minutes away. Each day Carol would pick up her granddaughters from school and take them to the local community center for their swimming lessons. It was Carol's favorite part of the day and something she always looked forward to.

Soon after Carol had decided to move away from her partner, her daughter informed her that they were going to sell their house and move thirty minutes away. Not knowing where she was going to live, Carol was not sure she would be able to maintain her routine of picking the girls up after school each day once they moved.

With the excitement of shopping for a new house, Carol's daughter mentioned to her one day that some of the homes they were looking at had mother-in-law quarters and how fun it would be if only Carol could move in with them. Carol's plans to move were unknown to her daughter at that point, and she was quick to inform her that she was planning on moving away from her partner at the end of that summer. You can guess how the rest of this story goes.

Carol was invited to live with her daughter and her family in exchange for helping out with the kids. Carol had manifested a beautiful home with a loving family by focusing on the absolute joy and relief of living in peace. She had her own room, her own bathroom, and a sewing/craft room nicer than anything she had ever had. If she had spent any time worrying about the how-to of manifesting what she wanted, she would have muddied the frequency that brought her exactly what she wanted.

All you need to focus on is what you want and how wonderful it feels to have it. Let the Universe figure out the how-to. It worked for Carol, and it can work for you too.

In the next chapter, I will teach you a bit more about how your brain works regarding hypnosis, and then I will teach you how to put yourself into a trance state to do self-hypnosis as you put your Personal Change Blueprint into action. You are learning to master the Law of Attraction!

*"Beware of what you set your heart upon…
for it shall surely be yours."*
Ralph Waldo Emerson

Chapter Twelve
Preparing for Self-Hypnosis

I teach self-hypnosis to many of my clients. Those who have listened to the hypnosis recordings I make for them ahead of time find it relatively easy to slip into a hypnotic state when doing self-hypnosis. This is because their brain is already wired to go into the state of hypnosis. Those of you who have listened to the hypnosis recording referenced at the beginning of this book will also find it easy to slip into a hypnotic state on your own. If you have not listened to the recording referenced at the beginning of this book at least four or five times, please do. It is to your advantage to be familiar with the structure of a hypnosis session and be wired to go into hypnosis before you practice self-hypnosis. You can find the link here https://debbietaylor-author.com/free-audio01.

What Does It Mean to Be *In* Hypnosis?

Before giving you the instructional process of doing self-hypnosis, I would like to teach you more about what it means to be *in* hypnosis. There are as many definitions for hypnosis as there are hypnotists to ask.

My very generic definition is this: "Hypnosis is a profound state of deep relaxation with a targeted focus." That is not a bad description, but if you have ever seen a stage hypnosis show, then you know those people on the stage are not really relaxed—or are they?

I remember when I first started learning about hypnosis. It seemed very mystical, and getting hypnotized seemed like something only "other people" could do. I was sure I had never been hypnotized, even though I had no idea what it meant to be hypnotized.

Hypnosis is a natural state of being, one that we all go in and out of several times each day. It has a lot to do with brainwaves. If you have listened to the hypnosis recording I provided, you will recognize the beginning part referred to as *the induction*. The induction is where I relax you from head to toe and then do a countdown from ten to one. The intention of the induction is to slow your brain waves to the theta state. This is the state associated with hypnosis. Understanding more about the different brainwave states will give you a better understanding of hypnosis.

Brainwave States

There are four stages of brain wave activity we are going to look at. From slowest to fastest, they are delta, theta, alpha, and beta. As adults, we experience each of these brainwave states throughout the day, depending on where we are or what's going on around us.

Delta is the slowest of the brainwave states, and as adults, if we are in delta, then we are in a very deep, dreamless sleep or in a coma. As infants, we are in the delta state for about the first two years of our lives (Laibow, R., 1999). Clearly, infants are not in comas, but they do not interact with their environment as we do as adults. Their little brains are like recorders. They observe and absorb everything in their environment. As they do so, they create millions of neural pathways based on what they are experiencing; the good, the bad, and the ugly. They do not yet have the cognitive ability to compare, contrast, or analyze what they are experiencing. They don't even have language skills yet, so they're not processing in terms of words. You know when you get older, and you recognize your parents in your behavior? This is where it comes from. Everything you experienced as an infant is recorded in your brain in the form of neural pathways and becomes the "norm" according to your subconscious mind.

Next up is **Theta.** This is my favorite because this is the brainwave state most often associated with hypnosis. Depending on what you read or who the author is, some authors identify the alpha state as more closely related to hypnosis. It is your ability to get into this state that allows clear and open communication between your conscious mind and your subconscious mind as you practice self-hypnosis.

As children, we evolve from the delta state to the theta state at around age two and have access to delta and theta exclusively until we are around six or seven. Theta state is fun! It's where we combine reality and fantasy, not yet having the ability to discern between the two, so it's easy to understand why kids at this age easily believe in Santa Clause, the Easter Bunny, the Tooth Fairy, and so on. Again, children at this age are not interacting with their environment the way we do as adults. They are recording, observing, and absorbing everything in their environment free from the filters of analyzing, comparing, and contrasting.

As adults, we go into this theta state at least twice each day and sometimes more. We always go through the theta state, right as we are waking up in the morning and right as we are falling asleep at night. This is why I recommend doing your self-hypnosis first thing in the morning. You are already so close to that theta state that it's easy to get right back to it.

Around the ages of six or seven, our brains evolve into the **Alpha** state. This is a big deal because, for the first time, we have the ability to analyze, compare, and contrast. This is the birth of the "conscious" mind. Up until this point, we have been operating only from the subconscious mind, in a state of hypnosis, you could say. All of a sudden, the idea of a jolly fat man in a red suit flying around the world in a sleigh, delivering presents to everyone in one night is preposterous. Before our brains evolved into the alpha state, it made perfect sense. All the programs and all the neural pathways that have been created from birth to this point remain active, unchanged until you consciously access this vast warehouse of the subconscious mind and update your programs. What beliefs and values did you acquire as a youngster that are in direct opposition to what you believe today?

Once we evolve into the alpha state, we are able to process information in a more sophisticated manner. We can do higher-level math problems, we are more socially aware, and the world takes on a very different quality than in previous stages of development.

Our brain development takes another leap into maturity around the age of twelve as we enter the **Beta** brain wave state. Over time the beta brain wave state continues to refine its development into low, middle, and high beta brain wave activity. This is where we spend much of our time as adults as we manage our hectic and sometimes chaotic life schedules.

The Critical Faculty

The conscious mind and the subconscious mind work in tandem, thank goodness, but there is an invisible wall separating them. This wall is referred to as the critical factor or the critical faculty. This wall is very thin and easy to "soften" for those who are very visual, imaginative, creative, or artistic. For those that are analytical or linear thinkers, this wall is a little thicker. It is this wall that has kept your conscious mind from communicating clearly with your subconscious mind to create permanent change in your life.

For example, your conscious mind *knows* that you want and need to stop snacking each night while you're watching TV, but until you get that message to the subconscious mind, the habit mind, not much is going to change. The momentum of the subconscious mind will win out every time. Remember, the conscious mind only contributes 1-5 % of what's going on compared to the 95-99 % of the subconscious mind.

Hypnosis is the process of relaxing you to the point that your critical faculty, that invisible wall, dissolves, and your conscious mind has a clear path to the subconscious mind via the imagery of your words, and voila! That's how you create the new habit of being a non-smoker, or how you find it easy to eat healthy food or to create other habits by choice. This is how you program yourself to make change. All you have to do is relax yourself to the point of reaching the theta state, and then review the imagery and the emotions of how you'd like your life to be. This is how you communicate with and rewire the subconscious mind and how you master the Law of Attraction. You can create anything you want. The sky is the limit.

*"As soon as you start to feel differently about
what you already have, you will start to
attract more of the good things, more of
the things you can be grateful for."*
Joe Vitale

Chapter Thirteen

Self-Hypnosis with Your Personal

Change Blueprint

Once you have completed answering all the questions in your Personal Change Blueprint, you are ready to put yourself into a hypnotic trance and review your Personal Change Blueprint while doing self-hypnosis. Start by reviewing the answers to all eight steps a few times, and then prepare yourself to do self-hypnosis. The self-hypnosis process outlined below will be very familiar to those who have listened to the MP3.

1. Find someplace where you can get comfortable and where you will not be disturbed. If you have a recliner, great! If not, sit on your bed with your back against the headboard and your legs stretched out. Or just sit in a comfy chair. I don't recommend laying down because I don't want you to go all the way to sleep. You may find it helpful to use an eye mask to keep the room nice and dark.

2. Begin by taking in a deep, deep breath. Hold that to the count of three, four, or five, and then gently release. Do this two more times, making each inhalation a little deeper than the one before. At the completion of the third exhalation, bring all your focus up around the top of your head and begin to relax your scalp, your forehead, your eyebrows. Think about all the little muscles around your eyes and your mouth and notice how they begin to soften with relaxation as you release any tension or tightness anywhere in and around the face, the neck, the throat. Follow that flow of relaxation down into the shoulders and let it cascade over the shoulders flowing gently through the arms, all the way to the hands,

releasing any tension or tightness from the fingertips.

3. Now, bringing your focus back to the larger muscle groups of the upper back and chest, notice how those muscles begin to soften with relaxation as you feel the warmth of that relaxation beginning to melt down the spine. Follow that warmth as it moves into the shoulder blades, down into the rib cage ... flowing all through the middle back, down into the lower back, through the pelvis, and into the thighs.

4. Feel the release of any tension or tightness all through the thighs as if it were simply evaporating through the pores of your skin. Follow the flow of that release through the knees, into the calves, all along the shins, through the ankles, and into the feet as you release any tension or tightness right through the tips of your toes. You're doing beautifully.

5. There are two ways we relax—physically and mentally—and you have just completed the process for physical relaxation. For mental relaxation, I want you to count down from ten to one, visualizing yourself walking down ten steps into a beautiful garden, or perhaps you are in an elevator going down

ne floor after another after another. Or perhaps you are on the beach. As you look at the wet sand, you notice that with each number you count, you can see that number as if it were etched into the wet sand. As those waves gently roll in and dissolve the numbers right before your eyes, you feel yourself falling deeper and deeper into relaxation, deeper and deeper within yourself as those waves gently roll out. Count slowly, rhythmically, and feel yourself dropping deeper and deeper into relaxation, deeper and deeper within yourself with each breath you take.

6. Once you have reached this state, it is time to review all the information you wrote down in your eight-step Personal Change Blueprint. It does not matter if you change the order of the material in your blueprint. It does not matter if you forget a detail here and there; you will be doing this again the next day. If you think of information that would have been a great addition to your blueprint, add it! Be mindful and use language that creates the imagery of what you *do* want if you add something new. Review the information as if you were

watching a movie of your new life story. Review it a few times.

7. Once you have completed the review of your Personal Change Blueprint a few times, you are ready to bring yourself back into your environment, back into normal waking consciousness. This is an excellent time to review the main idea, your outcome, one more time as you begin counting from one to five. Take a deeper breath with each number you count, start wiggling your fingers and toes to kick up your circulation a bit. On the count of four, take in a deep, deep breath and gather all that beautiful energy as you exhale on the count of five, opening your eyes. Give yourself a minute or so to acclimate back into the world.

8. Congratulations! You just completed a thirty-minute hypnosis session in about ten minutes. The more often you practice self-hypnosis, the less time it will take to get into the trance state and the quicker you can do your self-hypnosis each day.

Follow this process every single day; make it a habit. It is this repetition that creates new neural pathways in your brain and aligns the frequencies of your conscious mind with the frequencies of the subconscious mind. This is the secret to mastering the Law of Attraction by aligning the once competing frequencies coming from your mind. This is how you manifest abundance in all areas of your life. The secret has been revealed.

Common Questions About "Doing" Self-Hypnosis

I want to answer some questions you may have about the self-hypnosis process. I have been teaching self-hypnosis since 2008, and the following questions are the most common questions I am asked.

Q1: What is the best time of day to do my self-hypnosis, and can I do it more than once each day?

Because we go through theta as we wake up each morning, I typically recommend doing your self-hypnosis first thing in the morning. However, if you are one of those people who wake up bright-eyed and bushy-tailed, and you hit the ground running, then morning is not the best time for you. For you, I will recommend doing it in the evening between dinner and bedtime but not necessarily AT bedtime because I don't want you falling asleep in the middle of it. It's okay to drift in and out of sleep, though. If neither of those times works for you, choose a time in the middle of the day when you can take a break, clear your mind, and find someplace to be alone. You may find that mornings work best on the weekends, and evenings work best during the week. Experiment with it and find out what works best for you.

All in all, first thing in the morning is preferred. You can do self-hypnosis as many times throughout the day as you want, but never while driving. If you find that you are falling all the way asleep when doing self-hypnosis, then make yourself a little less comfortable the next time. Sit up straighter, put the lights on brighter, and put your feet on the floor.

Q2: Where should I do self-hypnosis?

It's easy to create the right environment in which to do your self-hypnosis. You'll need somewhere to recline or just lean back a bit. If you have a recliner, great, otherwise adjust the pillows on your bed and perch yourself up there. Turn the lights down low, take your shoes off, and put your feet up. Close your eyes or use an eye mask if you like. If you have pets, either let them onto your lap, to begin with, or put them someplace where they will not bother you. Use earbuds or headphones if you are piping in music or if you've made a recording of your Personal Change Blueprint. It's common to drop a degree or two in temperature when meditating or doing hypnosis, so have a throw blanket handy.

Q3: How do I deliver the information in my Personal Change Blueprint once I'm in the hypnotic state?

You have several choices regarding the delivery of information from your Personal Change Blueprint. After you have completed all eight steps to your Personal Change Blueprint, I encourage you to read over the information several times. Eventually, you will notice a pattern to the questioning, making it easier for you to remember what comes next. My preference is for you to review the information before you do the self-hypnosis and then remember it, think of the story it's telling. It's okay if you remember things in a different order than you wrote them. Just think of it as a story - your story, your movie, and you get to make it any way you want.

You could also make a hypnosis recording for yourself. This will take longer to listen to than if you just go over the information from memory, but unless you are in a big hurry, that is not a problem. We tend to think about 80% faster than we speak, so listening to a recording will take more time. You could also have someone you know make the recording for you. Some of us do not like the sound of our own voices, so if you want to listen to a recording, but you don't like the sound of your own voice, you might consider having someone else record it for you.

Another option is to summarize your Personal Change Blueprint and put the information on an index card. After you've finished the induction, simply give yourself the suggestion that in a moment, you're going to open your eyes to go over your blueprint, but that you will stay in a nice deep state of relaxation the whole time. If you've ever seen a stage hypnosis show, those volunteers on the stage have their eyes open and are very active, but they are still in hypnosis. Opening your eyes in hypnosis does not necessarily take you out of hypnosis.

Q4: How many days should I stay on the same subject?

Repetition is the name of the game when it comes to rewiring your brain and creating new neural pathways. I recommend staying on one subject for ten days to two weeks before going on to the next. You will most likely start to notice changes much sooner than that, but it's important to reinforce your Personal Change Blueprint details over and over. It's like practicing a new song on the piano. You have to practice several times to get good at it. Just because you get it right once doesn't mean you can stop practicing. You want the details in your Personal Change Blueprint to be deeply embedded in your subconscious mind so that your conscious mind and your subconscious mind are sending out the same frequency.

Q5: What if I miss a day?

No problem, get back to it when you can. If you're doing self-hypnosis in the mornings and you forget one morning or just don't have time, go ahead and do it later in the day or the evening. Remember, the beauty of self-hypnosis is that you can complete an entire session in ten minutes or less. The more often you do it, the quicker you will align your frequencies, the quicker you will master the Law of Attraction.

"Start telling the story of your amazing life, and the Law of Attraction must make sure you receive it!"
Rhonda Byrne

Chapter Fourteen
Conclusion

The first book I read on Law of Attraction was *Ask, And It Is Given: An Introduction to The Teachings of Abraham-Hicks* by Esther and Jerry Hicks. I was so excited to read the book and start manifesting everything under the sun. But the promise of "Ask, and It Is Given" fell short for me, as it does for many. Despite my best efforts and no matter how many times I *asked*, what I asked for wasn't showing up. And yet, I believed with all my heart that the Law of Attraction was real. I read every book I could get my hands on about the Law of Attraction, and I watched every YouTube video Esther Hicks ever posted. I even went to one of her live seminars in Portland, Oregon, a few years ago.

It wasn't until I became a certified hypnotist that I began to put the pieces together, which led to the development of the Personal Change Blueprint. I read *The Biology of Belief* by Bruce Lipton. He explained how we are only consciously aware of 1-5% of what we do each day and how it is the subconscious mind, the 95-99%, truly running the show. That was the missing piece. I finally understood why I was not receiving what I had been asking for. This was a game-changer for me, and I know it will be for you too.

We manifest every aspect of our lives, whether we believe it or not. We can't *not* manifest. I was recently chatting with a woman who was telling me how hopeless her relationship was. Her partner was just not behaving the way she thought he ought to. She proclaimed to be well versed in the workings of the Law of Attraction, but when she told me she was certain that she didn't manifest this relationship, that she would never choose this for herself, I knew her understanding of the Law of Attraction was faulty. Like many people, she was under the impression that manifesting only applies when you are intentionally trying to manifest, and it only applies to the good stuff.

We manifest everything in our lives. I can hear the arguments: "I would never manifest this abusive relationship!" or, "I would never knowingly manifest this lousy job, or this drug addiction, or this depression!" And that is my point exactly. None of us would knowingly manifest these unwanted things, but when most of your vibrational frequency comes from the subconscious mind, you don't know it; it's subconscious.

I have given you the tools to change the subconscious programs that have kept you living a life of manifesting by default. Now you have the tools to manifest by design, to master the Law of Attraction. In the words of Maya Angelou, "Do the best you can until you know better. Then when you know better, do better." Now you know better.

My most sincere wish is that you have a new understanding of the Law of Attraction from reading this book and that you feel a renewed sense of joyfulness at the possibilities before you. You are not broken. You have never been broken. You have simply been living your life by default, and now you can begin living by design—your design. In the words of Abraham, "There is nothing you can't be, or do, or have."

Appendix A
Your Personal Change Blueprint

You can download the eight-step Personal Change Blueprint PDFs here https://debbietaylor-author.com/free-blueprint-pdf or grab a notebook and write each of the steps listed below on a blank page.

Step One – Your Payoffs and Your *Now* Statement

Step Two – Crafting your Outcome for Exactly What You Want

Step Three –Your Evidence

Step Four – Imagery Associated with Your Manifestation

Step Five – Sounds Associated with Your Manifestation

Step Six – Physical and Emotional Feelings

Step Seven – What Change Does for You

Step Eight – Positive Influences

- Relationships
- Career/Finances
- Health
- Self-esteem
- Spirituality

References

(Laibow, R., 1999) Medical applications of neurobiofeedback. An *Introduction to quantitative EEG and neurofeedback* (pp. 83-102).

Mastering the Law of Attraction

Your Personal Change Blueprint

Debbie Taylor

https://debbietaylor-author.com

503-312-4660

Available to speak at your next event.

Go to https://intuitivelifecoachllc.com/

Mastering the Law of Attraction for Financial Wealth

Your Personal Change Blueprint

Scheduled for release Fall 2021